Jean Tsushima



Malmaison - London
22nd February 1974

# SPEAK FOR YOURSELF

## The Life of a Speech Therapist

# My Life and My Work Series

**Accountancy** *Taste for Accounting* by Peter Reynolds
**Advertising** *One Off* by T. E. Johnson
**Architecture** *Living Dimensions* by T. W. O. Carter
**Armed Forces: Navy, Army & Air Force** *All the Queen's Men* by Norman King, Richard Lawson, Dick Pierse
**Art · Painter & Teacher** *A Painter's Diary* by Francis Hoyland
**Author & Writer** *The Ring of Words* by D. J. Hall
**Banking** *Wealth of Interest* by J. B. Pickerill
**Child Care** *Children in Jeopardy* by Joan Lawson
**Dentistry** *Chew This Over* by Matthew Finch
**Divine Ministry: Anglican, Roman Catholic & Methodist** *Rev* by Stephen Hopkinson, John Foster, Ray Billington
**Education Services** *Beyond the Classroom* by J. M. Hogan
**Electrical Engineering** *Making Electric Things Happen* by P. L. Taylor
**Farming** *Down to Earth* by Donald Knight
**Hospital & Community** *Medical Social Work* by Helen Anthony
**Hotel & Catering Industry** *At Your Service* by J. Morel
**Housing Management** *Real Estates* by Prudence Baker
**Journalism** *Dateline: Fleet Street* by Owen Summers & Unity Hall
**Law** *Let's Make it Legal* by John Malcolm
**Librarianship** *Books are for People* by James Dearden
**Marketing** *A Consuming Passion* by Martyn Bittleston
**Mechanical Engineering** *Of Men and Machines* by George Stephenson
**Medicine** *I Swear by Apollo* by P. T. Regester
**Merchant Navy** *The Dustless Road* by S. J. Harland
**Mining Engineering** *Mines and Men* by Tom Ellis
**Prison Service** *Prison People* by Nicholas Tyndall
**Publishing & Bookselling** *Books are my Business* by A. W. Reed
**Radio & Television** *The Informing Image* by Rodney Bennett
**Retailing** *Can I Help you Madam?* by Marian Aitken
**Scientific Research** *Why Research?* by Sir Ian Wark
**Secretarial Skills** *Take a Letter Please* by Mona Tratsart
**Speech Therapy** *Speak for Yourself* by Betty Brown
**Statistician** *My Statistics are Vital* by Madge Dugdale
**Teaching** *And Gladly Teach* by Margaret Miles
**Theatre Management** *Beginners Please* by Elizabeth Sweeting
**Women Police** *The Gentle Arm of the Law* by Jennifer Hilton
**WRNS** *Never at Sea* by Vonla McBride

**My Life and My Work Series**

# SPEAK FOR YOURSELF

## the life of a speech therapist

by Betty Brown, M.C.S.T.

**Educational Explorers · Reading**

*First published* 1971

*isbn:* 0 85225 736 8

*Published by Educational Explorers Limited*
*40 Silver Street, Reading, England*
*Set in 'Monotype' Bembo and printed in Great Britain by*
*Lamport Gilbert Printers Limited, Reading*

CONTENTS

## *Also by Betty Brown*

with Laurence Ives, Dip.Ed.Psychol., A.B., Ps.S., M.Ed.

'*The Re-education of a Dysphasic Adult—an experiment in co-operation between a Speech Therapist & an Educational Psychologist*'

The British Journal of Disorders of Communication, the Journal of the College of Speech Therapists,

Vol. IV, No. 2, October 1969

# FOREWORD

It is customary and appropriate in work of this kind to take all possible steps to protect the confidential nature of the professional relationship. I have attempted to safeguard the anonymity of the people concerned by witholding identifying names and place names. But I have given them no fictitious disguise. There is no person described who has not existed, no incident recounted which did not happen and no conversation recorded which did not take place. This is because I believe that it is only by a faithful record of fact and feeling that one can represent those who wish, above anything else, to speak for themselves.

This account is offered in acknowledgment of the strength of those wishes and of the work of those who try to realise them.

Betty Brown

# ACKNOWLEDGMENT

*The Author and the Publisher gratefully acknowledge the kind help and advice given by*

THE CHAIRMAN and COUNCIL
OF THE
COLLEGE OF SPEECH THERAPISTS

*and are indebted to*

GRAEME McCAIG

*for the drawings which illustrate this book*

# AUTHOR'S PREFACE

When you have been practising a profession for some years it becomes increasingly difficult to recall accurately why it first appealed to you. At this point in time I cannot write about speech therapy without being aware of all the richness and warmth that are the result of being involved in human communication. The identification which the schoolgirl once felt for the speech handicapped child has given way to a much truer recognition of what this handicap may mean to the child and his whole family. The quick response of the healthy to the stricken, speechless adult has been replaced by a realistic knowledge as to how the inability to communicate can affect all aspects of a person's life.

The instinctive admiration felt by the student for the spirited child and plucky adult has given way to a tempered and profound respect for children, parents and individual people who struggle with buoyant courage to transcend the limits of their faulty communication systems. The pleasure in language has been deepened and intensified by learning something about its development, by being exposed to the many ideas as to its manifestations and its use. It is no longer possible to separate the initial attraction from the developed devotion.

But it seems to me that a job which has remained so lively and so stimulating for so many years must have as much to offer the young student who wishes to find out about life as it does to the mature adult who wants to make use of experience.

Speech therapy will attract those people who, out of a very

varied population, have the common link of an interest in the way people communicate and a desire to help the handicapped to communicate more effectively. As it involves adjustment and readjustment to one person after another throughout the working day, it is not for the academic who wishes to pursue a speciality to the furthest point of which she is capable. It will appeal predominantly to those who are responsive, emotionally sturdy and to whom communication is something to be valued and cherished.

Responsiveness shows itself early, other qualities are more difficult to predict. For most of us the choice of a career comes much too soon. We cannot be sure enough of our own reactions to know how we will stand up to other peoples' demands. We cannot be sure whether our interest will last and whether we have the emotional stamina to cope with the needs and demands of handicapped children and adults.

Fortunately emotional stamina, like so many useful qualities, tends to develop with use. Coping with difficulties is a great confidence builder so long as you can cope to good effect. But the initial commitment must always be something of a gamble. For the development of a therapist is necessarily the development of a person.

# I

## 'FIND YOURSELF SOMETHING TO DO, DEAR'

THERE ARE SOME PEOPLE who move up the school with their eyes fixed upon careers in medicine, teaching or architecture. They are often a source of envy to the undecided because certainty is always so compelling. I was not one of this number. Not only could I not convince myself that there was a particular niche for me to fill but nobody else appeared to think that there was any one special direction in which I should be elbowed or propelled.

By the time I reached the sixth form I was just such a person as career talks are designed to influence. I dutifully viewed myself as a social worker, infant teacher or librarian according to the prevailing model. I also produced a few counter fantasies of my own. There were the engaging visions of the woman surgeon with the surest scalpel, the finest Hedda Gabler of her generation or the barrister whose eloquence saved from the gallows innocent man after innocent man.

Such fantasies are a necessary defence against the daily revelation of deficiency ('Must work harder at the more routine aspects of the subject' . . . 'must take more pains to be accurate' . . .) But fantasy can widen the gap between the almost possible and the extremely likely. So I appeared to be heading for an exit from school without having established an entrée elsewhere.

Consequently I was encouraged to try for University entrance with the object of reading English. This seemed to be a possibility within my reach and one which satisfied some of the more romantic aspects of my character also. I could picture myself wandering through the cloisters discussing Shakespeare or Chaucer and alternating this with hours spent drifting down the river in a punt propelled by some outstanding undergraduate. I still tend to have unrealistic ideas about university life in spite of having eventually achieved it after about fifteen years and then on an enormous campus in the Mid-West of America.

I decided to attempt my university entrance undeterred by the knowledge that I had got as far as choosing a subject but had not considered the harsh question: 'What then?' To a young woman contemplating spending three years in an environment where the men outnumbered the women 'What then?' could afford to look after itself.

My dreams of academic life were shattered by a dramatically fractured limb which meant a spell in hospital and then a long period of steady attendance at the out-patient clinic. By the time I was ready to get back to work my classmates had far outstripped me. Moreover my enthusiasm for university life had somewhat faded. My musings had taken a more medical turn. I had also discovered a wish to do something useful for somebody which was, I suppose, the direct result of so many people doing useful things for me.

This image of utility, or perhaps service, did not blend easily with that of the English scholar or the white hope of the Old Vic. So I occupied myself in a rather desultory manner while waiting for my ideas to reform themselves or for something to turn up.

At this point I was given a bundle of career leaflets by a conscientious teacher and one of them was on speech therapy. And that was it. Seen through the imaginative eye it appeared to combine all the essential elements of medicine, teaching, drama and general utility which I was looking for. So I went home and told my family that I was going to be a speech therapist and everyone was very surprised because no-one had ever heard of it.

At that time speech therapy was very little known and there were only four places in England where it could be studied. All of these were in London. The profession was only just starting to become unified under the newly formed College of Speech Therapists. This had been set up as an examining and regulating body to try to ensure high standards of professional training and practice. Until the formation of the College, work had been carried on by individuals of devotion and resource who had become aware of the needs of the speech handicapped and were prepared to make considerable efforts to promote their welfare.

This had led several workers into the field of training and the schools of speech therapy founded by them necessarily reflected the ideas and aptitudes of these devoted and energetic women. Some showed strong leanings towards medicine and attached their schools to hospitals. The school to which I was admitted was the Central School of Speech and Drama originally founded by Elsie Fogerty to encourage the study of speech in all its aspects. There were then three courses, Stage, Teacher and Therapy.

Although I could hardly have foreseen it at the time, I was to have a long and continuing association with the Central School both as a student and then as a member of staff. I shall always count this as one of the blessings of my life. Not only was speech therapy, my chosen subject, given a new dimension by its association with other aspects of speech, but I was able to work with some of the most outstanding people in the whole field of speech, and exposure to giants is always a bonus.

My choice of, and my allegiance to, the Central School reflect my own particular bias and interests, and doubtless others would write with equal enthusiasm of their own establishments. There was rather more difference in the training schools then than there is now, and each had a very distinctive flavour. But because the courses were new and evolving they were not as well integrated as they are now. In fact, they were more than somewhat fragmentary.

Our basic subjects were Anatomy and Physiology, Psychology, Phonetics, Normal Voice and Speech, and Speech Pathology and Therapy. To these were added a number of shorter courses in specialised subjects, and they all had to be brought into relationship with each other by the efforts of our tutors. At the Central School very considerable emphasis was placed upon the voice training of the individual student. It was assumed that the speech therapist must be able to make a pleasing sound, to demonstrate all aspects of the speech function and to be clear and articulate in conversation. This still seems to me to be a reasonable assumption.

After three years of study and of practical work we were presented for our qualifying examination. There were papers in each subject studied, plus the ordeal of the practical examination. Here the student must be observed treating patients by two examiners from the College in what is somewhat unrealistically suggested to be a normal treatment situation. Every time I go out now as a College examiner I am reminded of my own ordeal.

The situation does not change very much. One has studied the case histories from A to Z, one has read all the works published by the examiners in the hope that if not impressed by one's words they may at least be confounded by their own. In the end all anxieties boil down to the simple prayer that one's patients will just turn up. However great one's clinical proficiency one cannot demonstrate it without a patient. And never is affliction so widespread among the clinical population as on examination day.

Adults who have attended with exemplary diligence throughout the term suddenly become afflicted with agues or decide to pop off to the seaside for a holiday. Children who have been sent away the week before with beautiful new 's' sounds lose their teeth like hailstones between one session and the next. It is always the same and no student will ever believe that her situation is not unique.

I passed this ordeal of initiation like so many other students before and since and was duly admitted to the College of Speech Therapists. My diploma was delivered by a friendly but curious postman. 'L.C.S.T. Now what would that be?' 'Licentiate of the College of Speech Therapists'. 'Oh, well. And the best of luck!'

WE THE COLLEGE
OF SPEECH THERAPISTS

do hereby admit

____________________

a LICENTIATE of

the College of Speech Therapists

this 19th day of November 19

Given under our common seal

*Chairman of Council* [illegible]

*Secretary* [illegible] *Date* 16th December 19

# 2

## 'I CAN SAY THE . . . THING'

### *Speech Therapy in the School Health Service*

I APPROACHED MY FIRST JOB with mixed feelings of pride, competence, excitement and inadequacy which must be very common. What a pleasure it was to be able to make one's mistakes in decent privacy after three years of being supervised and assessed. To be sure my knowledge was rather less deep and less broad than I had hoped but perhaps I could remedy this before too much harm was done and too many people found out. It was really splendid to be able to follow the whole treatment through from start to finish. There was the interview with mother, the speech assessment, the treatment and finally the discharge.

This whole sequence is rarely seen by the student. In fact it is not generally realised that few students see much progress at all. This is not entirely due to their own ineptitude. In order that they shall have plenty of clinical variety they are moved about a good deal. This can be a blessing if one is stuck with an unsympathetic therapist supervisor or a dull clinic. But it is very discouraging for everybody if you have to leave a patient just as you are getting to know him or he is starting to make progress.

Another unfortunate and depressing practice is that of keeping chronic patients on at the speech clinic to provide student fodder. No student is going to feel too happy about her chosen profession if she keeps seeing patients who have been treated for six or seven years. There may be patients who should be seen by a speech therapist to prevent deterioration rather than promote improvement but in my opinion they should be treated by staff. A student needs encouragement and the best kind of encouragement is success.

I certainly remember the patient who achieved normal speech while under my care and the fact that I recall him so clearly shows that this was a rare student phenomenon. The child in question had been unable to pronounce many consonants but in other ways he was a bright, competent little boy. The answer to a speech therapy student's prayer in fact. He went on steadily from strength to strength and sound to sound until I was driven to seeking out my supervisor.

'Ronnie has now established the "r" sound and he can control all the others in spontaneous speech and I don't really know what I should do next.'

'It sounds as though he is ready to be discharged.'

'DISCHARGED?'

Ronnie had not been available, needless to say, on the day of my practical examination.

I went out into the field with a certain amount of knowledge as to how children acquire speech and this was of great importance. But I found that I knew very little about the way in which normal, school-aged children spoke to each other. Present day students of speech therapy are required to do a good deal of observation in nursery and infant schools, so there is far less danger now that they will regard any articulate child of four as a kind of infant phenomenon.

I hastened to repair my ignorance by visiting schools and calling on friends and relations who had suitable offspring. It was important that I did find out because my appointment was to the school health service of a large county borough and I was, as the quip has it, 'responsible for all the defective speech among the school population'. I worked as one of a team headed by the principal school medical officer and he or his assistants were responsible for referring children to the speech clinic.

I had plenty of freedom to carry out my treatment and discharged the patients when I thought fit. I was free to arrange school and home visits and to organise my sessions as I wished so long as I kept the authority informed of my movements and projects. In fact I was treated in a manner that was extremely reasonable for a person who was responsible and specialist trained but inexperienced and newly qualified. Some of my friends were not nearly so fortunate. They had many more restrictions to contend with including having their patients actually selected and discharged by the medical officers.

Unfortunately there is still a considerable amount of variation throughout the country as to the extent of the speech therapist's responsibilities and nowhere more than in the School Health Service. Some restrictions have caused a great deal of resentment in speech therapists who are genuinely concerned to give the best service available and feel that they can best decide how this should be done.

On the other hand the public must be protected from individual team members who carry out their own projects without regard for the rest of the service. The school medical officer has the school population in his care and should know what is being done by all the members of his team. It is probably the flexible chief who gets the best work out of his team not by surrendering his authority but by knowing when to use it and when to let the spirit of the case take over from the letter.

It would be a great deal easier for both sides if there were more senior posts, well paid and responsible, for speech therapists who could direct and support the more junior workers. Unfortunately not only are the good jobs lacking but so are the therapists to fill them. In some parts of the country the shortage is so acute that the newly qualified are asked to take on jobs that are very demanding and very isolated.

The demands can be risen to in an amazing way but no speech therapist thrives on isolation. The College of Speech Therapists tries to overcome this by arranging area meetings and conferences. These are extremely valuable but a monthly discussion group cannot replace the student colleague who was always there to give suggestions, sympathy or just praise.

I had no-one else in my area and so I learned fast but not fast enough. I learned which children needed care most and why, but even this is a much more difficult decision than might appear. I was confronted with all the members of the school population who had not acquired fluent, articulate speech. Some had minimal problems and some very severe difficulties indeed. Some had developmental delays and some had wild deviations. I probably saw most of the classic speech disorders among children though I did not necessarily recognise them all at the time.

Part of the process of professional growth is to see, much later, the significance of something one has been looking at for a long time. I must have left undone a vast amount through ignorance but then I also attempted a good deal from ignorance too and this was not always unsuccessful. It can be an advantage not to recognise the impossible.

I suppose that a child's mastery of speech is his greatest achievement and really it is an incredible process that changes a little bundle of reflex activity into a creature who can understand the thoughts of others as expressed in speech and respond by expressing his own. This mastery of the sounds, words and symbols of language is achieved by normal children in three years.

Basically the organs we use for speech are designed for survival. The tongue, lips and jaw are for chewing and swallowing, the larynx for shutting off the lungs from the feeding tube. A child with a speech problem may have encountered difficulties in the basic functions of the speech mechanism too. Indeed, some brain damaged babies reveal this in their first cries. These have been shown to be different in quality from the cries of healthy babies.

A professor of speech pathology with whom I worked in America told me, with a becomingly apologetic air, how he conducted his research into babies' cries. He would descend on a ward of sweetly sleeping babies with his recording apparatus, waken them with a little tweak of hair or flesh and record the resultant fury. He would then slip away leaving a ward full of

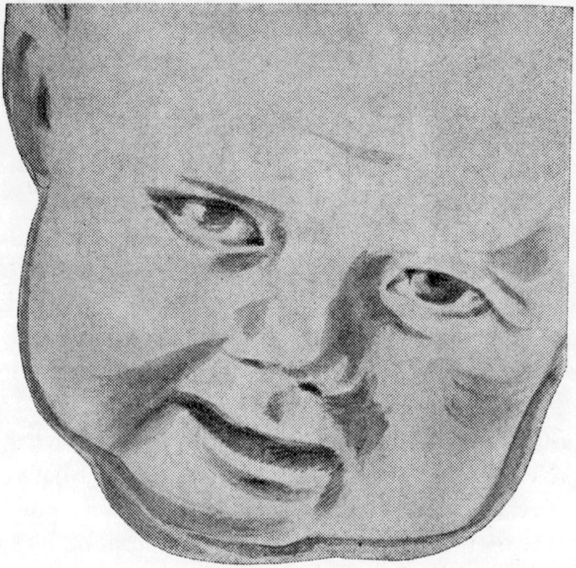

outraged babies to be pacified by the nursing staff. I wonder whether distant memories like these still lurk in the minds of children who become resolutely silent in the presence of a tape recorder.

The deaf infant will at first cry normally and will go on to babble and make other sounds so long as these are directed by physical pleasure or need. At the stage where the normal infant's sound play becomes influenced by the sounds of others, those of the deaf baby will disappear. For once sound is present it becomes modified and shaped by the speech of the mother. From her the baby learns words. If he is left on his own without stimulation he will not acquire speech so rapidly or so well. A child who is insecure will not have the incentive to communicate or experiment.

We know now that the quality of a child's language and probably his thoughts are very dependent upon the kind of stimulation he is given at home. If he says 'Bus' and the mother says 'Yes, bus', his words have been reinforced but not extended. If she says 'Yes it is a bus and it is going all the way to London' he has not only gained more words to imitate but more ideas to think about. His own character and intelligence will, of course, make a great deal of difference too. An intelligent child will learn more words in less time and combine them with other words in fresh ways to explore and develop his thoughts.

So if any child does not speak normally and at the normal time one must look for the cause in his own basic abilities and in the behaviour and attitudes of those close to him. One must find out what is lacking, what has gone wrong and then set about seeing whether things can be put right or whether the child must be taught to compensate for them.

A child may be unable to pronounce a certain sound because he cannot hear it, because he cannot distinguish it from similar sounds, because he cannot make the correct movement or because he is emotionally insecure and needs to cling to babyish patterns of behaviour; and those are only some of the causes. I can remember two young brothers, the first could not say 's' because of a cleft palate that had only just been repaired, the second because he had imitated his older brother.

Both learnt quickly to correct their pronunciation but with

different handling. The little boy with the cleft palate was very proud of his achievement and confided to me 'Now when he (the surgeon) asks me to say sixpence, I can say it. So he might give me one'. I incorporated this remark in my progress report to the surgeon and was pleased at his acknowledgement with the P.S. 'I have made a note about the sixpence'.

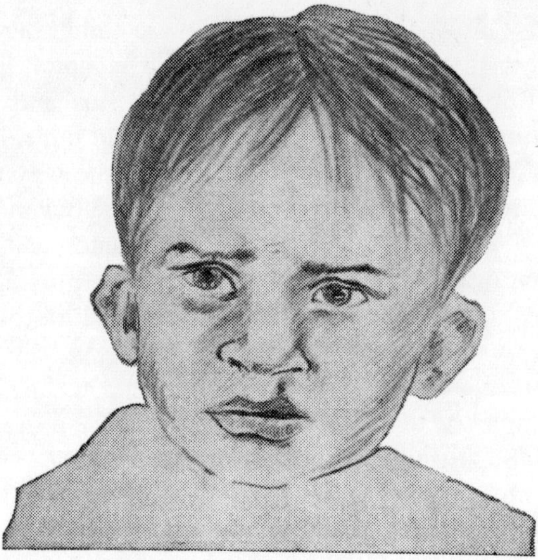

With so many things to consider it is very important not to rush into treatment before careful examination and observation. I remember seeing a small boy with delayed and distorted articulation at the time when psychological theories concerning speech were at their most prominent. The mother/child relationship was fraught with danger and many traumas to be expected in connection with oral gratification. I never met Raymond's mother as she would not accompany him to the clinic.

This of course made it much easier to pursue my own theory. If ever there seemed to be a disturbed child it was Raymond with his muttered inarticulate speech and abashed, embarrassed air. Indirect treatment with plenty of reassurance and creative activity was obviously just the thing for him. Mercifully after about three weeks I remembered to look in his mouth. It was then I discovered that he had no teeth.

The only comparable experience I had to this one was on arrival in the States when I was asked to supervise a student working with a very young and highly nervous little boy. The student was putting him through a series of stern tongue drills which was doing nothing for his confidence or their relationship. So I suggested that perhaps something less direct might be more helpful. I received an answer both reasonable and bizarre. 'But Mrs. Brown the only course I have taken is in articulation therapy so articulation therapy is what I have to do'.

We do have to spend a lot of time teaching children how to make sounds and it is important that they enjoy it. Why otherwise should they try?

It is difficult for a young child to realise why he should alter his speech as long as people know what he means. If the words are changed by his faulty sounds he may have more incentive. For example, if he says 'DAMN Mummy' instead of 'JAM Mummy, and gets a smack instead of a treat. But if he asks for 'ithe tream' instead of 'ice cream' he will probably get what he wants. Some people try to force a child to say a word correctly before giving him the thing he is asking for. But this is a bad practice. It can make the child unhappy and resentful. No-one can know how difficult it is for him to speak clearly so it is wisest not to assume too much. It is very difficult to change one's speech habits. One of our foremost speech therapists suggests that adults who think it is simple should try producing the sound 't' every time they normally say the sound 'k'.

So children must be induced to come over to our side by plenty of imaginative handling by the therapist. We are still sadly short of attractive clinical material and far too many of our cupboards are filled with sad old toys and books. Our motivating devices are rather sparse too, paper stars, drawings and of course the speech book. The speech book is likely to be with us for as long as children need to practice at home and with the present limited number of clinical attendances possible for each child this will be a long time.

So out of every speech clinic in Britain go the speech books, laborious records of the acquisition of sounds. Some of them are charmingly illustrated with drawings, or pictures cut out and stuck in by the children. The same illustrations tend to occur. 'Sammy the Snake' must have been hissing away all over the country for the last twenty years. His shape and his sound are far too propitious for him to be easily abandoned but I can't help wishing he would find a little friend to take over for a while. Even in the States I found him, green and curly, proudly displaying his 'new' sound 's'.

One little boy, Geoffrey, took particular pride in his speech book as well he might because it was a splendid record of progress from a few sounds to clear articulate speech. It was taken regularly to school to show teacher who had contributed very much to Geoff's progress by her interest. But one day the little boy arrived in tears. 'Why Geoff, what's the matter?'

'Miss, I've lost my speech book.'

'Never mind, I'll give you another one.'

'But Miss, I'll have to go back to the beginning again now.'

My room was situated in the main school clinic immediately on top of the dentist's. This had some advantages in that we could get together to discuss the effect of dentition on speech or tongue thrust upon dentition. It had very considerable disadvantages though, particularly on extraction day. Some pale and bleeding child always seemed to emerge just as I guided an especially nervous child up to my room for a soothing speech session. The room itself was quite cosy once you got inside. Indeed it was a little too cosy to be comfortable in summer.

It was not a very attractive room but it became very colourful and interesting by the time the children had brought me coloured pictures and pinned them up at their own eye level. I also acquired some interesting odds and ends for display like some plasticine models and a few curtain hooks that one of the children found he could spare quite easily. It is important that a speech room should at least look cheerful and friendly because many of the children are very nervous and easily intimidated.

A particularly nervous group is the stammering one and stammerers ranked high among my clinical population at that time. The severity of this symptom can vary from easy repetition to severe blocking with silent agonising struggle. People are easily embarrassed by stammering because they do not know how to behave or cannot behave as they should, which is naturally. They never know whether or not to prompt the stammerer and this can be difficult. It is usually wiser not to, because you may give the wrong word which is maddening. Or even if the word is correct the stammerer may feel a sense of defeat at not having achieved it for himself.

Bernard, aged nine, was a great struggler and I tried hard to get him to substitute a more relaxed repetition for his explosive utterances. One day he told me that he felt badly because all the other boys in his class were to have speaking parts in the nativity play but he had not. I spoke to his teacher and found, as I expected, that it had been a mistaken kindness on his part fearing to embarrass the boy. He immediately gave Bernard a speaking part but it was not the best one he could have had. It would have been easier if Bernard could first have said a few unimportant words among the crowd before speaking out on his own.

But I could hardly keep butting in so I rehearsed Bernard in his role of shepherd trying to ensure that he made his announcement of the star in the east as easily as possible. On the day of the play Bernard entered splendidly on cue and started with the vital piece of information about the 'st st st'. He was not doing badly and would have weathered it I am sure had it not been for a helpful child in the front row who volunteered 'Star'. Bernard's tongue was freed but the mood of the nativity play was shattered as he glared at the offender and roared 'I can say the bloody thing'.

The repetitive stammer may be the most obvious but the silent struggle is the most painful, and one child, Eric, who behaved like this used to worry me very much. He had had a very unsettled early childhood with no real home and now, at eight, he was living in a small institution for deprived children. He had little cause to trust anybody and certainly he did not seem to trust me. We moved very cautiously into our relationship and it did seem after a few months as if he was growing a little less inhibited and the struggling aspect of the speech was less in evidence.

I decided that I must get in touch with his teacher and find out how things were at school. This meant a first approach to the head master which gave me some feelings of trepidation. This particular head master was known to be a very outspoken man and I could well imagine his answer, 'I don't know what you are wasting our time for. He has been going to see you for three months and he is still stammering'. But I bravely wrote and shortly had an answer.

'At first I noticed no improvement' (gloom). 'Now I observe that Eric smiles more frequently, volunteers answers to questions and takes part in all class activities. Not only is his speech improved but he seems much happier in every way'.

That head master certainly made one speech therapist happier. He had shown me that this therapy business was not a myth or a confidence trick but that a child could be helped to communicate better and through that would become happier.

We were all warned as students not to become too involved in the problems of our patients but I later dropped that particular piece of instruction, at least in that form. People have to come to terms with their own feelings in their own way. As clinical judgement grows experience becomes easier to handle. Also, if one is fortunate one has learned from other people, or preferably from one other person, that one is loved and needed. The patient must not be asked to demonstrate this to you. But at first there is, almost of necessity, too much emotional involvement. It is only gradually that one learns how to create the kind of therapeutic relationship which will free the patient from his dependence when he himself is ready to be freed.

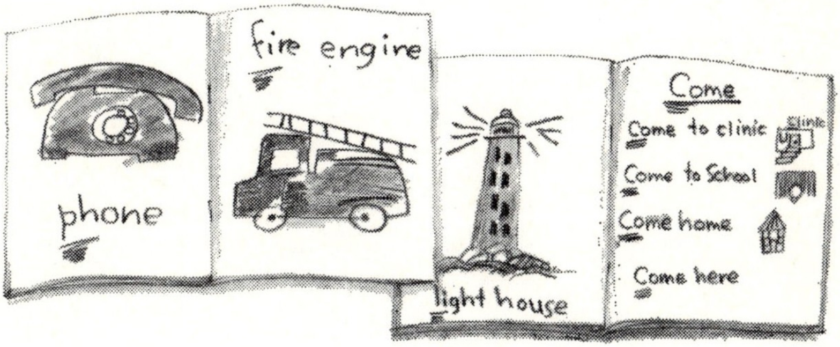


This process was shown to me most clearly by an adolescent stammerer. He was a delightful person but with very strong feelings of inadequacy related to his speech and general lack of confidence. At first he appeared with incredible punctuality and treated all my utterances with extreme respect. The opportunity of discussing his feelings weekly and at length with a young woman was probably as much help to him as any exercises in speech fluency.

As he progressed he became a little more casual. He was never late but he stopped coming with such desperate alacrity. He did not cease to respect my opinion but he started to challenge it. And then finally he expressed the change for himself. My therapist's soul delighted but my womanly heart suffered a pang when he said brightly.

'You know, I used to look upon Tuesday as the one day in the week that mattered, the only thing that kept me going. But now, well, it's just another day'.

# 3

## SPASTICITY, SPEECHLESSNESS AND SPIRIT

### *Speech Therapy with the Cerebral Palsied*

DURING MY YEARS with the School Health Service I had become increasingly interested in the cerebral palsied or spastic child. Cerebral palsy is the name given to a group of conditions in which the control of movement is impaired due to brain damage. Spastic has caught on with the general public as a rather snappy term and so tends to be used indiscriminately by the lay person for the whole group. The child who is born with this condition may have to be taught to make all the movements which the rest of us acquire naturally and without effort. Speech is particularly difficult because it involves so many small movements which need to be finely co-ordinated.

The condition of cerebral palsy is not a progressive one but, as the child grows, his difficulties become greater unless he has been treated. Now we like to start working with babies, helping them to feed and to carry out all the basic movements on which speech can later be built. The older a child is the more difficult it is to build the easy movement patterns which he needs for skilled activities.

I had seen very few spastic children during my training and had not developed any special feeling for their problems. But as soon as I started meeting them as individuals in my clinic it was impossible not to become very much involved. My first spastic patient was a very appealing and delightful child which may have made a difference. But I think I must have responded anyway. Any speechless child pleads silently for our help but particularly the spastic who has so little outlet for expression and communication.

My own interest coincided with and was undoubtedly stimulated by a considerable increase of interest in both the medical and educational fields. Physiotherapists were starting to develop a much greater variety of techniques as well as a much more thorough and systematic approach to treatment. So it behoved the speech therapists to do likewise.

I was lucky in meeting a very devoted and able home teacher in my area who taught me a great deal about what the children's difficulties meant in terms of everyday living. Then, as I got to know more parents of spastic children, I saw the continual problems they were attempting to solve every day not only to help their children develop to the greatest extent possible but just to get the whole family along with the minimum of distress.

I became involved with the newly formed parents group which was able to put all sorts of pressure upon the local authorities to get treatment and schooling for their children. Local authorities have considerable powers but they also have many demands. It is easy for an official body to disregard a section of the community that is not causing trouble. But when parents really get together and make demands they tend to get what they want and particularly when they have shown how much they themselves are prepared to work for their children and all other children like them.

We had our social activities too. There was a hay picnic in the summer in the field of a farmer who had a spastic boy. And our first Christmas party was a joy with the decorations that the children had made in school, the carols they had practised in speech clinic and a wonderfully benevolent Father Christmas portrayed by a local doctor, himself the father of a spastic boy.

These are the fringe benefits that add enormously to one's professional life. This is the kind of classless society where everyone is genuinely involved in helping each other and where '*Honour done to one is a joy to all*'.

I said earlier that ignorance could be a help in that it prevented one from recognising the impossible. In my early enthusiasm I did not know what was possible and so of course I achieved success and failure rather indiscriminately. So when I learnt about John who had never had any treatment and was now sixteen and speechless, I thought that no harm could be done by trying; and I trundled off to see him on my bike twice weekly

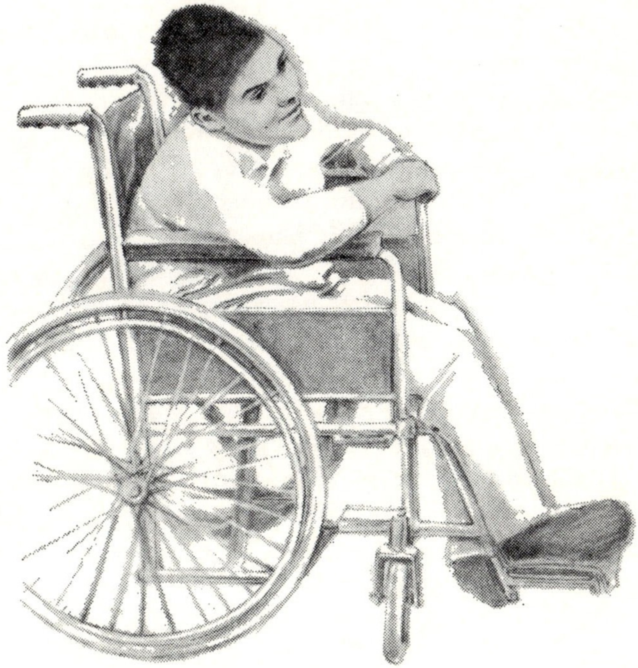

after clinic, undaunted by the impossibility of the task. Now I know that harm can be done by trying. Hopes can be cruelly raised and frustrations increased.

But in this case no damage was done. John's parents were practical, sensible people who had lived too long with their son to expect miracles. And as this is a true account I cannot record that any miracle ever took place. But positive benefits did occur. John did not learn to talk but he gained another friend who provided some interest and variety in his life. His parents gained a little help in how to feed him more easily. And I became known as a speech therapist who was willing to have a go which meant that many more spastic children were referred who could benefit.

One thing I learned from this association which I shall never forget. John had a friend, Bob, who lived down the road. He was a Mongol boy of about twenty and he spent his days at the local Occupation Centre (as it was then called). In the evenings and at weekends and holidays he would drop in to visit John. They would sit together in a silence broken occasionally by some observation of Bob's. He was not embarrassed by his friend's silence any more than John was embarrassed by the lack of content in Bob's remarks. Each recognised and supported the other. They communicated and they valued each other's company. And this, after all, is the real stuff of friendship.

Sometime after this I decided that while ignorance and enthusiasm were good starters they were poor masters. If I were to do anything to help these children I must find out more about them. In particular I must work more closely with the physical and occupational therapists to find the best way in which total treatment plans could be made. There were two possibilities, further training or a change of job. I had not succeeded in saving any money owing to a small salary and an uneconomical disposition so I opted for the latter. A post was advertised at a school for spastic children in Edinburgh. I applied for it and, in spite of being a Sassenach, was successful.

Edinburgh is a city which offers everything to the person brave enough to penetrate its austere majesty and the wraiths of mist that swirl about it. I walked into two major experiences at the same time—Edinburgh and cerebral palsy. The school was housed in a fine stone building originally a private house and now adapted by means of lifts, ramps and rails to accommodate its new population. The children were given every help towards independence in spite of their restricted mobility.

The staff consisted of the warden, matron, housemothers, teachers, physiotherapists and an occupational therapist and myself, speech therapist. The schoolrooms were large and bright, the physiotherapy room was very large and bright, the speech therapy room was bright and very small indeed. I say this without rancour. Speech was valued but space was at a premium. A child cannot walk without space but he can utter. Well, up to a point. Now that I have reached an age and position to command attention, I insist on all the adjuncts of my skill in the shape of tape recorders, language masters, audiometers and the space in which to house them.

At that time I had little except plastic feeding tubing and the largest mirror in the place to make up for having the smallest room. Oh, and a pair of plastic tongs which had been specially made for manipulating spastic tongues. These were bequeathed to me and I never had much success with them. The tongue is known to be an unruly member and it is certainly difficult to get hold of between two pieces of plastic. Fingers before forks and certainly before tongs. The child's own finger, suitably cleansed, or my own, wrapped in a sterilised finger stall in deference to the principles of hygiene, was found to be much more effective.

It is important to make the movement for the spastic child in the first place because he has no muscle memory to guide him, or rather he has only an abnormal one. So if one simply asks him to try to lift his tongue he will do it in the only way he can, which is abnormally. Most spastic children with severe problems are functioning at a reflex level with regard to speech muscles. That is, the actions that come most naturally to them are the primitive ones that happen to preserve life.

I mentioned earlier that the larynx is basically a valve which shuts to prevent foreign matter entering the lungs. It also closes at times of effort such as lifting something heavy. If this primitive reaction happens during speech it is impossible for the child to produce voice. Tommy was particularly afflicted in this way and it was very much at variance with his disposition which was sociable and charming. He loved to settle down for a good chat but I soon learned to get this over before treatment not after.

The effects of a long session of relaxation and easy vocalising could be entirely undone if one was thoughtless enough to fire a question at Tommy as he was leaving. As he recalled some interesting anecdote his interest and consequently his excitement would rise. This would precipitate a vocal spasm and we would both be trapped. Even if I became skilful in finishing the treatment session without this occurrence I never managed to avoid it in the corridor. It is not human to pass a friendly child like Tommy without a word of greeting and certainly it was not possible for him to pass any of us. Sometimes it was all right but if one spoke too loudly or suddenly the spasm would appear.

The most outstanding time it appeared was when we were both on our way to the puppet play. This was a project devised by the occupational therapist and myself for therapeutic purposes although we intended to entertain as well. Children with difficulties in hand control had made or were to manipulate the puppets and my lot was speaking the lines. Tommy was one of my stars. As we passed each other we both smiled and made as if to speak. I must have caught him on the wrong breath so to speak because the struggle commenced, mounted and went on. It seemed to last for about five minutes. Finally Tommy made it: 'Hallo', he said, 'I'm in good voice'.

I met Tommy again after a gap of fifteen years and was charmed to find that he spoke easily and without spasm. This visit was notable also for meeting Jean who had been a pupil and was now a housemother at a new school for spastic children. There were so many more that I would love to have seen, and heard, again.

You would get fond of these children anyway because they are fun and lively and you are working together. But you get more involved with them than with some of the other children because of the number of problems you have to solve together. Take feeding for example. I recommend this task to any speech therapist who is in danger of becoming too academic in her advice to parents. You just cannot know what a difficult and time-consuming business it is to feed a spastic child unless you have done it.

There is a line in *Paradise Lost* about offering someone something 'which he with spattering noise rejected' and that is a pretty good description of the feeding process with the spastic child. It isn't that the food cannot be put in. But in doing so a wave of spasm may be set up which results in the whole lot shooting back at you. The food stained figure holding a child's mouth firmly shut is a far cry from the calm, white coated professional speech therapist imparting to eager children the rules by which they learn to speak.

Sometimes one wonders how one got there. I was as fastidious as most young girls and can remember rushing round the corner to heave after seeing a man spit rather elaborately in the street. Little did I think of the pleasure I would gain from teaching a child to spit. It is a very necessary accomplishment. Try cleaning your teeth without spitting if you need to prove it. When children have inadequate breath pressure and immobile tongues their mouths can get very messy indeed. The final task of the feeding session was usually a good chase around the child's mouth for food particles. After this the occupational therapist

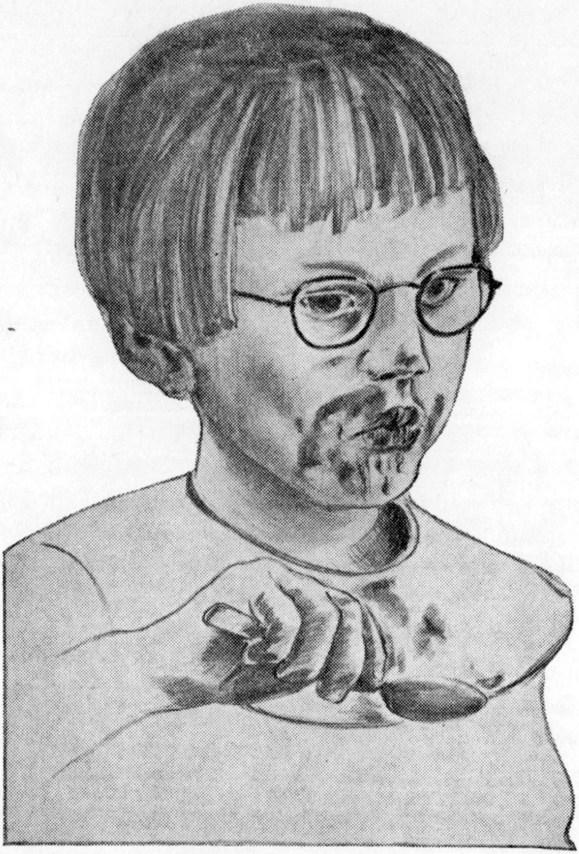

and I would repair to the staff room for our own lunches. But we never really fancied them.

Independence in feeding is of tremendous importance to the total independence of the spirit. It is very hard to detach yourself from your mother if she has to feed you well into adult life. Children longed to feed themselves except for the few who had unfortunately realised too early and too well that there is no point in doing for yourself slowly what other people can do for you fast. These children were nearly all conditioned to think this way by their parents before they came to us and it is an attitude very hard to undo.

It must be very hard for busy parents to leave the child to complete a task which may hold up the entire household for a great time. And of course, sometimes the effort is disproportionate to the achievement. That is why therapists are needed, early, to guide parents as to how much to demand of their spastic children. As one gets older this guidance becomes more practical and more easily accepted. As a friend of mine said in public: 'When it comes to helping parents there is nothing like a wedding ring or a few grey hairs'.

I can remember trying to hold one child back from taking her drink by herself through a straw. Her tongue and lip control were really not good enough and she was sucking in a great deal of air. I explained this to her but she answered me with equal conviction and goodness knows an equal case that if she could learn to do this she could take her mid-morning coffee at home without having to keep her mother from the many things she had to do.

When a child of eight puts such a point to you it must be respected. It shows the maturity that you are trying to help her achieve. So treatment so often becomes a compromise between what the therapist must do to improve the function of the mechanism and what she must concede to help the person live in dignity. Happily these things very often go together. The delight of therapy with the cerebral palsied is to see, not only their physical progress, but the personalities that are revealed as they gain independence. The joy of using speech for luxury purposes not just necessities is important indeed. I think I made one of the worst mistakes of my career when treating one of these children by not remembering this.

The girl in question was nearly sixteen and so would have to leave school that year. We were all determined to make her as competent as possible in the time we had. So she was on an intensive therapy programme in every area. In speech we worked on lip movements, tongue movements, sound production and combinations of them all. We worked hard and we worked to some effect.

But one day as I was getting the mirror out for her I saw the reflection of her face. The poor girl looked depressed and disconsolate beyond belief. And one could see why. To spend your time day after day in doing things that were always difficult, to be always working at things that were just beyond your grasp, was too much to ask of anyone and particularly of a girl of sixteen who might have been spastic but who had all the sensitivity and yearning of any other girl at that age. I put the mirror away.

'Do you like poetry? Because we are going to read some today'. We did. We read Yeats and de la Mare and Hardy and Housman. We read together and we read to each other. We ended up with *The Highwayman* accompanied by marvellous wind and storm noises. We were there for hours and I only hope it redeemed for her some of the weeks of struggle that must have seemed to her so purposeless.

Not all of the children would have put up with it so long. They were a spirited bunch, well able to stand up for themselves. This was a tribute to the school and particularly perhaps to its warden. It is bad enough for children to be handicapped. They should not be forced to become meek, docile, perpetually grateful.

One quip from a thirteen year old boy stays clearly in my mind. I had just about had enough of reminding him about his speech and he had just about had enough of my nagging. Finally

I said to him, 'Oh very well Billy, if you can't remember to speak more slowly and clearly, could you try to think of your audience as being hard of hearing and a little slow on the uptake'. It must have given him considerable satisfaction to look at me with one raised eye-brow (in itself a difficult achievement for a spastic) and to say with exquisite clarity, 'Naming no names?'

The acknowledged leader of the children had a fine spirit and had also done very well in speech. I was anxious to use him at a demonstration to be given to a large number of medical officers and other medical personnel who were visiting for the day. Demonstrations were the bane of everyone's existence. They were necessary in a teaching and research establishment where new methods of treatment were being explored. But they were time consuming and fraught with hazard.

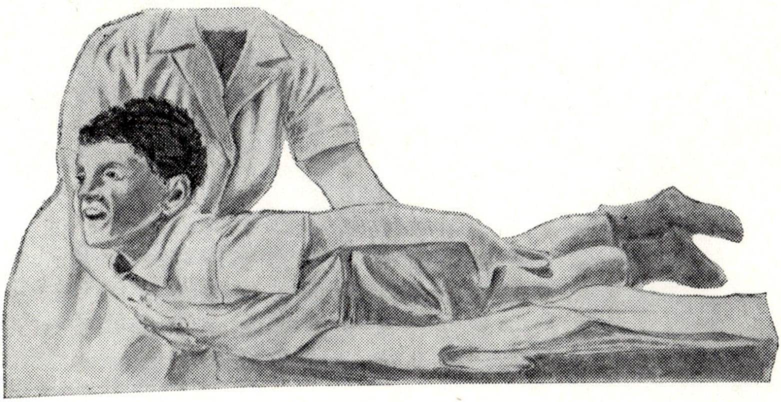

We all had our opinion as to whose was the most difficult skill to demonstrate but I will yield to no-one in my assertion that it is speech. In O.T. and P.T. they may not be able to produce the results they usually get but at least they do not have to contend with the child suddenly becoming tongue-tied just at the moment he is required to utter. To be sure our children were used to visitors and were rather chatty people on the whole. Some of them were quite capable of holding forth to a roomful of people if they felt in the mood. But you never could tell with demonstrations.

So I trapped this particular boy one day and obtained his consent to demonstrate 'if I can choose my own piece'. Unsuspecting and relieved I agreed. I had expected to have to bargain for much longer for this boy had many things to do always and the last demonstration had meant a day's release from speech and physio to get on with his car washing business. So my mind was set at ease about the demonstration which was the last I was to give before leaving Edinburgh.

I did not bargain for having to sit in front of my audience radiating good humour while a most vigorous reading was given from a book of Scottish history concerning a battle in which the valiant, hardy and resourceful Scots routed and demolished utterly the usurping, weak and cowardly English!

# 4

## THE WORDS THAT WILL NOT COME

### *Speech Therapy for the Stroke Patient*

I RETURNED TO LONDON to teach speech therapy and to work in a hospital department. The idea was to spend half my time teaching and the other half in practical work. The students would accompany me to the hospital to observe or assist. It all sounded very stimulating, which it was and easy to manage, which it was not. Those of us who have tried it know that in fact you are taking on two full time jobs.

Patients are there because they need treatment and not just as teaching material. They have a right to expect your time and care and that does not necessarily end at 5 o'clock. To a patient on the ward recovering from a stroke, or awaiting an operation on his larynx, the fact that you have a pile of student essays to correct and have been on the job all day is a supreme irrelevance.

But students need extra time too. They need to talk as well as to be instructed. Probably your best teaching is given to the student who will stick it out with you and end a long clinical afternoon with a cup of coffee at the corner café and a cathartic chat about the significance of the day's events.

I was doing a considerable amount of learning of course, as well as teaching, and nowhere more than in the area of adult aphasia. This is a condition where the ability to express one's thoughts or to understand the thoughts of others through speech is radically interfered with by damage to certain areas of the brain. This can happen after a stroke or an operation for the removal of a tumour or after head injuries. As the brain damage is selective the patient can think, and of course, feel. It is difficult to imagine a more humiliating condition for a mature adult, or a more disabling one.

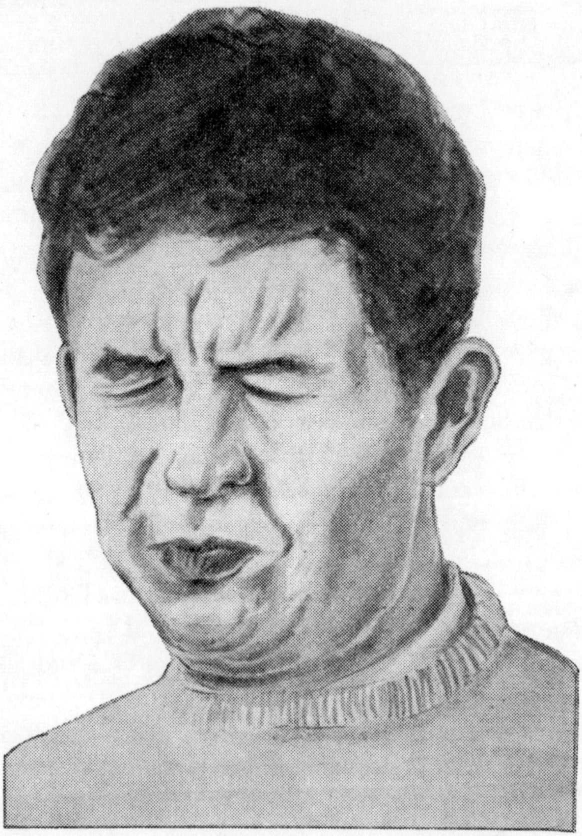

'I wanted to speak but I could not. I tried again but I could not speak. I thought to myself "What has happened to me?" I tried again but I could not and then I panicked. "What has happened to me" I thought to myself. "Oh, it's terrible, terrible" '.

These words were written by an aphasic patient after he had recovered some of his ability to communicate. After the initial panic he tries to think things out a little. 'I thought that I had had a blow on my head. This had hurt some, but not all, of my brain. For instance I could think quite well even if I couldn't speak or write. I felt I must appear intelligent even if I am not . . . then I thought that I might be still intelligent but I would be the only person who knew about it. I felt I was in prison through my own fault'.

Unfortunately patients' feelings of bewilderment and humiliation are so often made worse by the way other people treat them. It seems inevitable that people speak to the speechless as if they are mentally retarded or have become prematurely senile. Everything makes the humiliation worse. And there is the loneliness too. Very few of these patients can be admitted to rehabilitation centres where they can have company and some kind of social life. There are very few such centres and, such places as there are, are available to out-patients with physical handicaps for the main part. Many aphasic patients have accompanying paralysis of one side of the body but others are able to function normally except for speech.

It would not be difficult for friends to call on them and arrange activities which would break up the long day or evening. It is not difficult to communicate with an aphasic person especially if you have a common background. But although some people can do this easily others cannot and their defection is another cause of pain to the handicapped person. I suppose it is a healthy animal instinct that causes people to shun an afflicted member.

It could also be a primitive superstitious fear of the unknown. Neither have too much place in a society that aspires to progress.

But most often it is inertia and lack of thought. And this is sad. For while professionals are battering away at Government and local government departments to try to get more efficient provision for the needs of the aphasic much more could be done by all of us.

The task that faces some aphasic people is overwhelming. I worked with two young women, one of twenty nine, the other in her early thirties. Both had suffered strokes arising out of heart conditions. Both made good physical recoveries and were discharged home, totally speechless and with minimal ability to read or write. Betty had a husband and young daughter, Ivy had a husband and three young children.

The details of these women's lives became as familiar to me as my own. Together we learnt the names of every member of the family, the dog, the cat, the budgerigar. We compiled shopping lists, translated knitting patterns, exchanged recipes. We practised telephone calls with minimal speech to be used in emergencies.

'Baby sick'. 'House on fire'.

Ivy became particularly good at this and would often telephone herself if prevented from coming. 'Ivy'.

'Oh, hello Ivy, something wrong?'

'Yes, baby, doctor'.

'Oh, I'm sorry, is she bad?'

'No, better, doctor'.

'Oh good, well, I hope to see you Tuesday'.

'Yes, Tuesday, goodbye'.

Such conversations were models of information and celerity and doubtless many husbands would like the model more generally adopted.

By the time real communication had been achieved we were bound together by tears and trauma, gaffes and giggles. We had built up a system which used every remaining language asset. Both of them made considerable use of intonation. There could be no mistaking a 'No' of incredulity for one of admiration or one of denial. Both of them nearly always ended their early treatment sessions by the word 'Yes' said pleadingly and with great force. One could not ignore or misunderstand.

'Yes, yes, you will get better'.

And this was true and I believed it even though they never recovered their language to anything like the extent which they had previously known. But they recovered a great deal and they learnt to communicate with efficiency and charm, and with an ingenuity which was a continual pleasure and source of admiration. My role changed as they became more independent from a comforter to a teacher and finally to a woman friend, known for a long time and to be turned to in an emergency.

A natural advantage I had in working with Betty and Ivy was the common territory into which most women can enter fairly easily. But of course one never knows when one is going to have to learn up an entirely new subject for the patient whose main interest it is. Many an ill-informed speech therapist can be seen hastily scanning the football results before the enthusiast appears. One rather hopes that one is not going to have to rehabilitate a theoretical physicist or an expert on Siberian folk music, or that, if one does have to, they will have homely little hobbies like collecting match box tops.

My own knowledge and interests have been immeasurably extended by working with sophisticated highly intelligent aphasics from the world of the theatre, music and politics. This kind of experience is a bonus indeed for the work-a-day clinician. But it carries a high degree of responsibility also and is emotionally very demanding. Language means so much to these people. Their lives may have been spent in communicating ideas and such a life is now completely shattered until some way has been found of bringing the pieces together again.

One of the hardest workers I ever treated was an actor and writer who became aphasic in his early fifties. He always had something to explore, something to talk about or something he wished to have explained even at a time when his language was very restricted indeed. He would carry around with him copies of old acting scripts which he used to hold up in front of his face while travelling on the underground. Behind this screen he could mutter away practising making statements about what he saw around him. If he was overheard, his mutterings might be taken to be those of the enthusiastic Thespian conning his lines.

This man showed a very great deal of insight into the variability which all aphasic patients reveal. On a good day you can do a great deal of work and on a bad day you just can't. This may be a factor of the brain damage itself or it may be something brought about by language limitation. If one is unable to express one's thoughts and feelings adequately then one is so much at the mercy of external events and subjective impressions.

Sometimes you can help a patient to work through his feelings of depression and irritation but sometimes it is really better to divert him to some physical activity or relaxation which won't make so much demand on an irritated or tired nervous system. I can remember my actor patient coming into my room one day and simply saying, 'Sorry, no good today. Nice to see you but no good. Come back Thursday', and off he went to watch a cricket match or have a drink and I was in no doubt that he was absolutely right.

I do not mean to convey that it is only the well educated who value speech and language. They may use it for a greater variety of purposes but they do not have a monopoly. One patient I worked with had just started a small newspaper business when he had to go into hospital for a minor operation. Unfortunately while on the operating table he suffered cardiac arrest and only survived because of a great deal of emergency work by the operating team. During the time of the heart arrest there had been a stoppage of blood to the brain and consequent damage.

This man regained his speech very rapidly but he lost the power to read and write. He felt this loss very much. Not only was his business now in jeopardy but all the efforts he had made in the past to improve and educate himself seemed lost. People would now think that he was just an illiterate fellow who had never been able to read and write. He started to work with me with splendid stoicism but as he pointed out 'They call me a miracle of medicine but I wouldn't have minded being something more ordinary'.

Rehabilitating asphasic patients is not just a question of attempting to teach them to utter. It is the attempt to restore with them and to them their ability to use language to the greatest extent and in the most meaningful way. This restoration will be very much affected by the relationship that exists between you and the common ground you can establish. People talk best about things that mean the most to them. But then you have to have the techniques which will get language going in the first place.

It is fascinating to find the things that are retained. Nearly always the patient can recall some simple language sequences, the days of the week, number, songs. Singing is good therapy for nearly everyone. Frequently a patient can sing correctly a song that was popular in his youth, although he would not be able to produce the words consciously or by themselves. We tend to make use of this. Apart from the fact that it is rather impressive to visit a speechless person and leave him singing like a lark it is good for the patient to hear himself uttering.

Therapeutic devices can then range from singing, counting, copying, to complicated discussions and high level language activities. Douglas Ritchie wrote his book *Stroke, The Story of a Recovery*, to encourage other people and to help himself. His therapist told me when he started on the book and I thought it was a splendid idea and one which might well be emulated. So I mentioned it to my actor friend on his next visit. He replied amiably but quite unambiguously.

'Book eh, aphasia; jolly good luck to him. Personally, damn fed up, whole business'.

# 5

# NOISES BEAUTIFUL AND STRANGE

## *Speech Therapy with Vocal Disorders*

THE CLIENTELE OF THE SPEECH THERAPY DEPARTMENT in a hospital will vary according to the specialised nature of that hospital. In a neurological or rehabilitation unit the patients are likely to be preponderantly aphasic. In an Ear, Nose and Throat Hospital there will be many cases of voice disorder. A children's hospital will, of course, yield many of the same conditions found in the School Health Service but with a higher proportion of children with severe disorders or where there are difficulties of diagnosis.

The speech therapist in a large general teaching hospital, such as the one in which I worked for many years, will find that her patients vary according to the interest in speech displayed by the medical staff. It is usual for the speech therapist to be taken under the wing of a department which yields a high proportion of speech problems. This can be excellent, for the therapist feels that she belongs somewhere and receives support and stimulation from the staff of the department.

Speech therapists are usually more solitary than physiotherapists or occupational therapists who tend to work in large departments geared towards rehabilitation. Frequently the speech therapist is the only one of her kind and very frequently she is only a part-time member of staff. Many speech therapists hold several sessional appointments with the result that they are not in any hospital for long enough to become a real part of the establishment.

Among the many drawbacks to this arrangement is that of accommodation. Part-time workers be they psychologists, physicians or speech therapists have to cuckoo in other people's nests and a very uncomfortable business this can be. Hospital clinics are notorious for over-running their time and it is not unusual to have to wait, with several patients, outside the door at the beginning of the afternoon session while the morning occupant finishes off his work. Carefully timed interruption is one's only resource and this must be done with due regard to the importance of the person in occupation. Teaching hospitals are not very democratic institutions and the houseman gets more interruptions than the consultant.

I can recall many visits to the administration offices to point out the iniquities of the system but rarely was action forthcoming. The hospital was being rebuilt, replanned, reorganised, moved and there was not enough space to go round. This was certainly true and the speech therapist was not necessarily particularised though it sometimes seemed like it. We tended to blame our predecessors who, in their justifiable concern to get something started, were too abnegating about their requirements.

If you start off by agreeing to work in a cupboard you will still be in that cupboard in twenty years time and it will come to be accepted that this is where speech therapists work. It is worth driving a hard bargain to begin with. Fortunately one is never without weapons. After a doctor has suffered a series of vocal exercises going on with increasing power in the next cubicle while he attempts to take a case history, he is usually very ready to support your plea for a nice large room at the other end of the corridor.

It is important though not to be too isolated, for policy in this region, as in so many, is highly influenced by geography. A consultant working in the neighbouring clinic will be much more likely to get together for a case discussion than one who has to be visited at considerable distance and consequently by special appointment.

The hospital where I worked dealt with the question of how to administer the speech therapy department by making the speech therapist and her assistant responsible to a committee composed of a paediatrician, a psychiatrist, a plastic surgeon, a neurologist and an ear, nose and throat surgeon. Referrals for speech therapy came through any of these consultants. Like all administrative measures this had its cumbersome side but on the whole it worked very well.

SPRING. TERM. 1970.

| Patients Name. | Clinic 1. APHASIA. | Clinic 2 DYSARTHRIA. | Clinic 3 DYSLALIA. | Clinic 4. APHONIA. | Clinic 5 STAMMERING. |
|---|---|---|---|---|---|
| J. Osborne (Mr) | | | ✓ | ✓ | |
| Miss Flynn. | | ✓ | | | ✓ |
| " Grace. | ✓ | | ✓ | | |
| " Hill. | | ✓ | ✓ | | |
| " Innes. | ✓ | | | | |
| D. Day. | | ✓ | | ✓ | ✓ |
| Mr Ernest. | | | ✓ | | |
| Ivan Jones. | ✓ | | | ✓ | ✓ |
| T. Clayden. | | ✓ | | | ✓ |
| | | | | | |

There was no danger that an aphasic would be sent away untreated because the speech therapist was considered to work entirely for E.N.T. Patients were never referred directly to the speech therapist by an outside doctor and this is common hospital practice. It is frequently necessary for the patient to have a special medical examination of some kind and, even if not, some doctor has to take ultimate responsibility. Again, like many administrative measures the system works well or badly according to the attitudes of the people involved.

I don't think any speech therapist would be arrogant enough to dispute the necessity for a medical examination and referral. But difficulties can and do arise over diagnosis. Doctors on the whole know little about speech, its development and its deviations and are consequently not usually in a position to suggest lines of treatment or even to indicate where the deviation is occurring.

But there are some cases where the observations of both doctor and therapist must be co-ordinated very finely and most vocal disorders come into this category. The human larynx is a robust instrument in spite of the exquisite delicacy of its construction and it will take a good deal of strain. But the vocal cords cannot be expected to stand up indefinitely to repeated abuse. Many voice users whose jobs require sustained speech in unpropitious conditions come to the ear, nose and throat clinic with chronic or acute laryngitis. This may be a clear warning that the patient needs to keep quiet for a while but such warnings are rarely heeded.

The conscientious teacher or clergyman feels he must struggle on and so, in order to avoid inconveniencing others for a day or so, gives himself a thorough going voice disorder. Singers who try to sustain notes at a pitch almost out of range may start showing huskiness and fatigue. Actors designed by nature to play Feste who insist on playing Othello may also set up chronic inflammation of the vocal cords. Their voices will fatigue more and more rapidly and finally they will have great difficulty in making themselves heard at all.

I remember a woman who came to me with a history of recurrent voice loss. She was a member of the Salvation Army, forced to use her voice to attract the attention of people out of doors in all sorts of weathers and then to try to persuade them to listen to the gospel. Such a situation has all the components necessary for a voice disorder, difficult physical conditions plus anxiety. The uniform of the Salvation Army with its high collar tends to make for rigidity of posture and rigidity and excessive muscular tension are great enemies to good vocal production.

This woman responded very well to re-training and we built up her voice again steadily from a gentle easy tone to a good robust sound. The final stage was practice in singing and as the hymns of the Salvation Army are tuneful and infectious this was a very enjoyable part of the treatment. We were interrupted on one occasion by the E.N.T. registrar who walked in and gravely placed a penny on the table.

Voice troubles are not only found among professional voice users, for the voice is particularly vulnerable to emotional states and can by its behaviour give a very good clue to the underlying state of mind. People can lose their voices in states of anxiety or emotional conflict. One woman lost her voice following the death of her aged father in hospital. He had been senile and bed ridden for many years and she had tried hard to cope with him at home. Finally it became too much for her and he was taken to the institution where he died.

The woman took this very badly, and her guilt at having to send him away was intensified by his death. The loss of voice was a symptom of her inability to cope with her feelings and so obviously simple vocal exercises were not going to help her. A patient like this may be treated by either the psychiatrist or speech therapist depending on the severity of the underlying emotional conflict.

Such a patient is at one end of the scale while at the other are the patients whose voice problems are the result, not of misuse or of psychological difficulties, but of disease or injury to the larynx. Some patients are found to have malignant growths which necessitate the complete removal of the larynx. The surgeons who perform these operations are doing them to stop the spread of the disease and so they have to take away as much tissue as is necessary. But they try to reconstruct the throat in such a way that the patient can learn a substitute way of speaking.

A hole is made into the throat below the larynx and a breathing tube is inserted. The larynx is then removed so that there is now no longer any connection between the breathing apparatus and the mouth. Consequently air no longer comes up from the lungs, making sound by causing the vocal cords to vibrate. The patient can breathe perfectly well through his new airway but he is now totally voiceless. There is then a simple technical problem to be solved, namely how to provide him with a new vibrator.

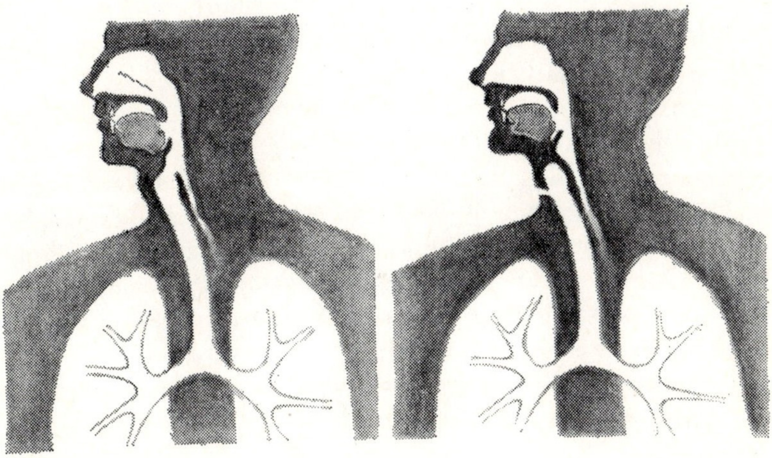

The most acceptable method for most people is pseudo voice or osophageal voice. Air is taken into the mouth and driven back in a belch. This belch is used to provide the underlying vocal note onto which the sounds of speech are added. The simple technical problem then is solved quite easily.

But human beings are not machines and a great deal of emotion is involved. The operation itself is a very severe shock to many and the resulting voicelessness can be terribly distressing. Moreover it is not easy for a patient to tolerate this crude start to voice rehabilitation. We are brought up in this country to hide our belches, not to produce them proudly. In some countries a good belch is a sign of gastronomic approval and it would be a great deal easier for British speech therapists if the habit could be adopted over here.

As it is the patient must not be allowed to feel embarrassed by the noises he is asked to make so the speech therapist sits there belching pleasantly and easily until he can be induced to imitate her. This is another thing one does not bargain for when considering one's future profession. Indeed it must be said that many speech therapists do not find it easy to treat the laryngectomised especially in the early stages.

At first there may be a lot of messiness with mucous in the throat which has to be fetched up through the new airway. Too much air swallowing can lead to all sorts of rumblings abdominal and other strange sounds. The patient and his relatives have to accept these things and so must the speech therapist. Indeed her whole behaviour must emphasise that these are unpleasant adjuncts that will gradually decrease and that the patient has not been rendered in any way repulsive by his operation.

Considered in general terms the whole business is daunting in the extreme. Considered in particular it is a wonderfully gallant and pretty efficient business. Every speech therapist has her story to tell of the degree of proficiency a laryngectomised patient can attain. We vie with each other in boasting of their attainments in using the telephone, in addressing meetings, even in giving lectures.

The best pseudo-voice sounds like a deeper and somewhat hoarser variant of the normal but it is not conspicuously abnormal and many a laryngectomised patient has been amused to be asked by a stranger if he is suffering from laryngitis. The road to this easy speech is taken by people of courage and the ones who succeed best are those who are stable, outgoing and with a good sense of humour. Such patients frequently form the nucleus of special clubs set up by speech therapists or patients where the laryngectomised can get together for mutual support and to give each other good practical tips.

Whether she sponsors such clubs or not the speech therapist always has her old friends among her former patients who will call on the new patients and show them that life can be full and good again and that speech is a real practical possibility. This is the most convincing reassurance that can be given for, as one patient wrote to me after such a visit, 'I believe you now'. I don't remember who his visitor was but it may well have been Micky. He was one of my greatest helpers though at the beginning he was as near suicide as a man can be.

Micky was only in his late thirties when he had to have his operation and he could not reconcile himself to it in any way. He was a publican and prized the welcoming, friendly atmosphere he gave to his cosy West End bar by the way in which he welcomed and talked to all his customers. It did not seem possible that he could ever achieve this with such a handicap and like all men of dignity he shrank from the thought of being an object of curiosity and pity.

There was no fear of that. He was basically a fighter and once convinced that the game was worth it he fought with everything he had got. I introduced him to a journalist who had had his larynx removed many years ago when he was much the same age as Micky and they got on like a house on fire. Micky made a good recovery from the operation and started to speak in record time. As soon as the voice got going he was back behind his bar, neat and dapper with a bow tie to hide the new airway.

He managed extremely well in ordinary conversation and only had to get assistance for the 'Time Gentlemen please' which is so rarely heard by the drinking public. Once established in his bar Micky was an enormous help to me. New patients were sure of a prompt visit on the ward or, even better, an invitation to drop round as soon as they were able for a double spot of cheer.

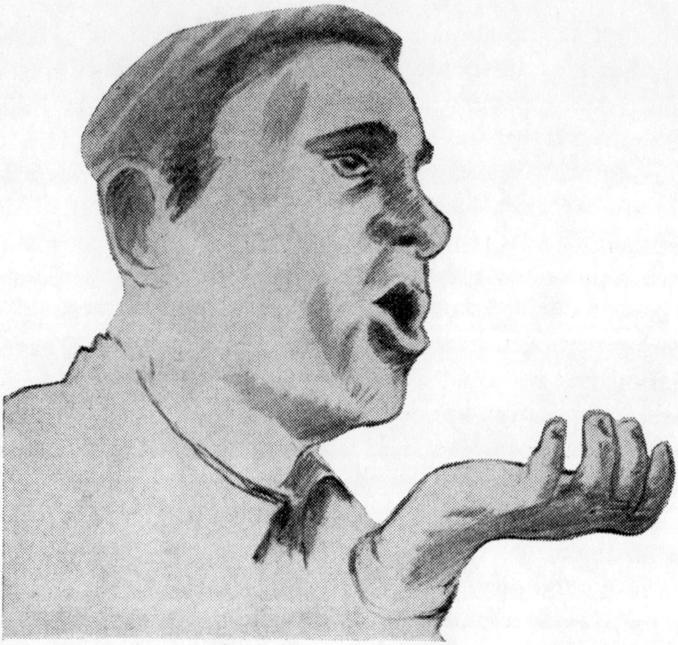

Micky's bar became a meeting place for quite a number of patients—'They hear us talking dear, and they don't know who's taking the micky out of who'.

Once established and controlled, the pseudo voice sounds warm and human with normal stress patterns though limited in pitch and vocal range. It is consequently much to be preferred by most patients to the mechanical sound that can be given by a battery driven vibrator. There are excellent vibrators on the market and they are invaluable for patients who have to have extensive surgery and so cannot achieve good pseudo voice. Sometimes a patient asks for a vibrator straight away.

I met one who had done this because he was a company director with many meetings to attend and this gave him a chance of getting back on the job more quickly and of coping with it with less fatigue. He used his vibrator very effectively and did not wish to learn pseudo voice. However one evening I was at a dinner party in his company when the vibrator suddenly failed. He was immediately transformed from a lively host to a silent member. It was a humiliating experience and we decided after that that it was worth trying to master pseudo voice to avoid such indignities.

One patient from Dorset had a rich dialect immediately audible even in the earliest stages of voice training. He was a splendid trier with implicit faith in the wonderful London hospital which had saved his life and he considered that he owed it to us all to become really proficient. One day his wife heard strange sounds coming from the bathroom and entered in alarm. 'It's all right' said the patient with dignity, 'I just thought I'd have a go at singing in my bath'.

Singing is not really a very practicable possibility though Harry had a better shot at it than anyone I have ever heard. He was in his late seventies when the operation was performed and had been a concert party entertainer singing songs at the piano. He reckoned that his voice was past its best anyway but there was still a bit of life in it.

In addition to singing he used to work 'living marionettes'. These are the kind where the performer puts his head through a hole in the curtain, suitably hatted, and then uses his hands to manipulate the diminutive doll bodies underneath. I was invited round one evening for a performance and have the most vivid memory of the little clown and soldier dolls dancing away, all chanting in pseudo voice.

It is easy, looking back, to recall the success of these people and forget the despair and the setbacks that they encountered during the process of rehabilitation. I recall one very charming and elegant man in the private wing who was almost totally unable to produce the requisite crude, belching basis. Progress came very slowly with staccato, uncontrolled utterance that fitted so ill with his elegant appearance and privileged style of life that I had real doubts that he would stick to it. The break through came one day when he was having a good deal of struggle which brought on a severe choking attack.

With an expression of the utmost distaste he vanished into the next room. I started to do a little experimental noise-making to see whether there was any other way which would help him to produce voice with less difficulty. I was working my way down the word list when I heard a voice behind me say quite clearly, 'If you're not careful . . . (long pause) . . . you'll get stuck like that'.

This man illuminated a rather hard and depressing clinic for me by later calling in on his way to Ascot. In his morning dress with elegant cravat he was a vision of the civilized man. The deliberate, slowly drawled speech in no way detracted from his charm and the impact on the newest recruits was terrific. While no one was quite naïve enough to think that a laryngectomy was an automatic pass to the Royal Enclosure, here was veritable proof there were no social restrictions if a patient did not wish for them.

By a splendid stroke of luck a woman patient was there who had had a very difficult time emotionally. She really hated the whole business which is, indeed, very hard on a woman. She feared that the operation had reduced her charm and limited her life to a very great extent and she frequently deplored her action in listening to her family and consenting to the operation. She was in middle age and a smart, fashionable woman who worked in a dress shop. This, like many other things, was no longer possible as it seemed to her, and there was nothing she wished to do instead.

As first she consented to try to speak but the rough, crude notes so repelled her that she refused to continue. She was prepared to visit me on a friendly basis but had no wish to speak. Fortunately for us both the surgeon was a great source of strength and support. Patients have great faith in their surgeons and they are right because in my experience not only do they work most skilfully but they are concerned to get the patient back into life and will do everything possible to promote his speech and his welfare.

The particular doctor concerned with this patient was prepared to play a waiting game, just as I was, until she was ready to accept herself and start to look ahead. She was just starting to do this when our visitor called. Already she was taking an interest in her appearance again and this was leading to a more active social life which was leading towards communication. I think that she would have persevered anyway but this beautiful figure before her was certainly no deterrent.

Once started this woman became a great ally and in her turn visited and inspired women who had the same fears as her own. She did even more. I had arranged to talk to the nursing staff about the laryngectomised and she volunteered to come and speak in my support. 'The nurses do so much for you when you are in and so ill, and then they never get a chance to see you when you are all right. So it will be nice for them to see how well I am'.

This was marvellous coming as it did from someone who had hated the operation and despaired of ever enjoying life again. And there was something for me too.

'I'll be glad to come and help you any time. Just give me a ring. I always answer the phone myself.'

# 6

## HOW CAN A STUDENT LEARN FROM YOU?

### *The Speech Therapy Training School*

THE NEW CLINICAL EXPERIENCES to which I was being exposed at the hospital were forced to compete for interest and attention with my new teaching duties. I had no teaching qualification and at that time there was none open to me. The Diploma of the College of Speech Therapists, in spite of its high standard, was not then accepted as a means of entry to any postgraduate course at a University or a College of Education. So my only assets in teaching students were the successful conclusion of my own student career and the clinical experience I had gained.

Once more I was in a situation where my enthusiasm was considerably greater than my knowledge. Looking back it appears surprising that I was not more daunted. This time I cannot claim to have been protected by ignorance of my task. It would be disingenuous to suppose that anyone would turn to teaching after some years of practising a skill without any realisation of the scope of the subject upon which that skill was based.

I accepted the post in my former training school because I liked the idea of trying to communicate to students some of the things which I believed, and had discovered, to be important. These concerned attitudes as well as information. I could not assess how adequately I was going to be able to do this but I had sufficient respect for the principal of the school and the director of the department to believe that, if they assumed me capable, then I might very well turn out to be so.

The principal, in particular, had an extraordinary gift for making one believe that anything was possible. This was just as well because the timetable I followed would have brought the strongest to his knees. Mornings of classes, tutorials and case discussions would be followed by precipitate journeys across London and then by long afternoon clinics. Evenings had to be devoted, however reluctantly, to preparation and marking. This left almost no time for further study.

I did become a little desperate whenever I had time to reflect on my precarious academic balance. Keeping one jump ahead of the students sounds well in anecdote but is uncomfortable in practice. My situation was beautifully illustrated for me one Easter when I was on a walking holiday in the Cotswolds. In a field in front of me was a large sow with about eight piglets. The piglets were sucking frantically at the sow's teats while she, poor creature, as frantically gobbled turnips. Where would it end, one wondered? Who would stop first?

It was difficult to complain about excess and pressure of work as the director of the department appeared to thrive on an even more demanding schedule which she had followed for twenty years or more. Also, like many people, I was capable of working fairly well under pressure because I could create enough energy by my own activity to replace some of that which I was giving out. A certain level of creativity can certainly be maintained this way. But not the highest kind.

The highest kind of creativity was not, however, often required from me in my role of tutor and junior staff member. It had to be positively suppressed for much of the time when a steady flow of mundane tasks had to be attacked or avoided according to their urgency and my mood. The worst and least avoidable of my tasks was the clinic rota.

Speech therapy students spend a large part of their student days in clinics. They must receive a variety of practical experience which means different clinics and different therapists to provide maximum learning. Our training clinics were scattered all over London and the home counties. This meant that in addition to trying to ensure equality of clinical experience one must also try to see that the number of long and expensive journeys was equally distributed.

Finally, one must allow, so far as was humanly possible, for the temperamental vagaries of therapist and student. The intuitive poetic streak of the introvert student might not be acceptable to the organised realism of the extroverted clinician. Or, of course, vice versa. After several hours of labour, despair and black coffee, I would present a rough draft to my superior who would point out some of the flaws and suggest I try again . . . and again.

Of all the duties from which I later graduated, none gave me more exquisite pleasure to relinquish than did the clinic rota!

Students were prepared for the College of Speech Therapists examinations as in my day and my responsibility for their success gradually increased during my years at the school. I met the students in lectures, seminars, tutorials and clinical demonstrations. The basic, straightforward lecture course was, for me, the most difficult of the teaching situations.

Most of us are capable of giving one good lecture upon a certain aspect of our subject. This is usually quite enjoyable for everybody because the cream of the subject can be taken without any necessity to get down to too much detail. But a regular teaching course comprises the basic facts about causes and conditions presented in the context of present ideas.

Students must be exhorted to read the literature, which means in fact, that they must be told exactly what book or article to find. Upon this base must be built the technical competence and psychological insights which will produce therapy. A considerable amount of repetition and redundancy appears to be inevitable. It is hard and devoted work to teach such courses in the way we would all like to teach them. Most fall a little short in some respect.

Many of us tend to vary between the idealistic 'they must learn to think for themselves' and the realistic 'they have to get a few facts into their heads somehow'. One cannot forget that one is training students to carry out a service as well as hoping to stimulate them to individual creative effort. One would like them to be capable of highly imaginative, deductive work but if they are not going to be in the top flight the teacher has a responsibility to see that they attain a certain level of straightforward clinical competence.

I was frequently more than a little remiss in giving students opportunities to take the kind of notes that appear to be essential to relieve their anxiety. This is simply because I prefer to lecture to faces rather than heads and pens. But every so often my conscience would compel me to undertake a session in which the whole lecture would be dictated slowly with headings and the minimum of fanciful illustration. One was then faced with the prospect of those words being reproduced by every student in every essay and examination paper.

The seminar, in which students participate equally with the instructor, is an excellent way to teach therapy. As well as exploring the literature and discussing the ideas contained therein, clinical techniques can be evaluated. The success of those seminars depends upon the willingness of the students to participate and the amount they are disposed to contribute. It takes some skill to conduct a seminar so that it does not degenerate into a sounding board for the opinionated few.

It is by no means the easy way out for a lazy teacher. Most of us have had the experience of rushing in to take a class during a busy period thanking heaven that someone else has prepared something, until it becomes apparent from the heavy blankness that each student has arrived with the same thought. But a successful seminar is a very good experience for everybody. There is real and active exchange of ideas and the level of comment and elucidation can be much higher than that reached in a series of statements from one individual.

Some groups of students very quickly integrate themselves into a lively but cohesive whole in which the individuals can express themselves freely but without too much disparity or hostility. Some groups never achieve this and remain a lumpish, uncoagulated class, each student only functioning well in an individual situation.

Opportunity for this individual function can be provided by the tutorial and this, again, can be a highly profitable occasion for both sides. I always enjoyed the tutorials that were built round case discussions. The student's clinical case book was produced and we both set out to explore what had been going on. Sometimes the cases would be those treated at an outside clinic and would simply provide a basis for a fairly generalised discussion. Sometimes the cases would be ones which I myself was supervising.

This meant a rather more pertinent and penetrating examination. Records have to be carefully scrutinised and the observation checked and supported. Above all, students must be helped to be as honest as they can be about what they are doing and why. Each student wants to present herself in a good light before her supervisor as well as to try to convince herself that something is being achieved. So one reads 'Mary seemed much happier in clinic today' and 'Mary brought her new book to show me' and 'Mary's mother said that she had been a very good girl this week'.

'And what exactly are you doing with Mary?'

'Well, I'm building up rapport, and . . .'

'Yes?'

'And I thought I would go on to letting her express herself by using paints or modelling clay'.

This might, of course, be perfectly relevant and apposite to the child's needs. Alternatively the poor student might really be saying:

'I don't know what on earth to do with this child and the only way I can keep her quiet is to let her play'.

The supervisor is only going to find out which version is correct if the student trusts her enough to relax her defences.

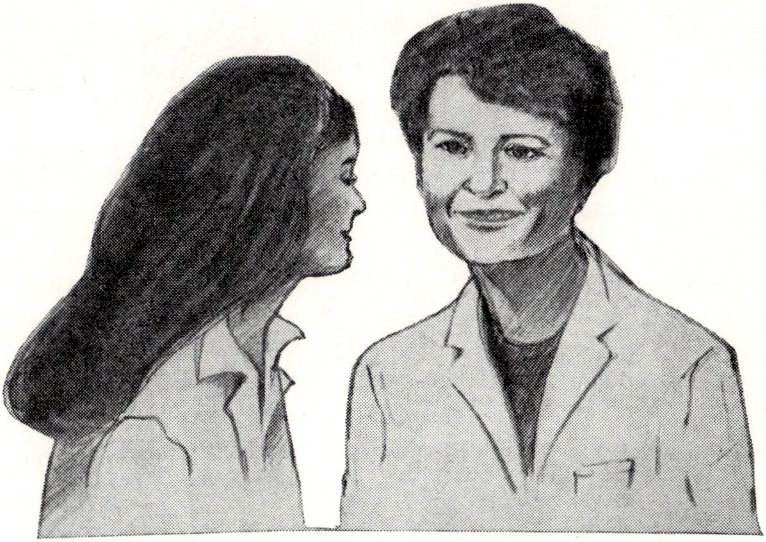

The tutorial may also be the place for good, practical advice.

'How is Mr. Jones getting on?'

'Well, actually I wanted to speak to you about this . . . only it's a little difficult . . .'

Mr. Jones is a stammerer of twenty-three. The student is an attractive girl of twenty-one. It isn't really so difficult.

'He wants you to go out with him' or 'He's asked you for a

date'—depending what side of the Atlantic one happens to be on.

'Well, yes'.

'If you don't want to go out with him, you can tell him that you are not allowed to have personal relationships with patients; and if you do want to go out with him, I will transfer him to another student'. Simple, but the looks of incredulous gratitude are a little disconcerting. Do they think that one does not know the occupational hazards? Or indeed that one is entirely immune to them oneself?

Clinical demonstrations are excellent ways to teach clinical techniques and reveal attitudes. Probably the best teaching situation is where students can watch treatment from behind a window that allows them to see but not be seen. The patient is told that they are there, of course, but he may be induced to forget about them. We had no such facilities when I started teaching and students were in the room during treatment.

Given good relationships all round this can work perfectly well but it can be difficult. Many patients do not like an audience . . . and some like one too much. It is still easier for everyone than the situation in which the student treats the patient in front of her supervisor. It takes a good deal of tact on everyone's part to prevent what the Americans call 'role confusion'. The student must learn and must therefore take responsibility but the patient must not suffer.

Nothing is easier than to reduce a student to confusion by interfering with her treatment and then step in to demonstrate one's superior skill. And nothing is less forgivable. The role of a student therapist is quite as difficult as that of a teacher therapist and it has to be played against a background of anxiety. The student is constantly being assessed and this assessment is directed not only towards academic achievement but towards personality development and clinical potential.

During the first year the student naturally tends to project on to you whatever feelings have resulted from her earlier experiences with figures of authority. So it may take time to achieve the good working relationship in which clinical teaching can take place. Unless this relationship is achieved the student cannot learn from you. One very intelligent student worried me very much by her apparent coldness and apathetic attitude. This seemed to suggest boredom which made me feel that I must give her more stimulation.

When the scope and depth of the patients' problems became apparent to her she would surely react with more interest. This was a perfectly reasonable premise and completely wrong. Far from becoming more at ease and absorbed the student became more and more withdrawn as I produced and demonstrated my patients with their variety of symptoms and needs. Eventually the poor girl broke down altogether and burst into tears. This was something of a relief to me because most women can cope with tears if they have to. We seemed at last to be getting to grips with the trouble.

I was confounded to realise that my demonstrations were making the girl feel more and more miserable because they emphasised the patients' needs. This made her increasingly aware of her inadequacies in being able to meet them. She had enough intelligence and sensitivity to be already acutely aware of the patients' state and her self distrust and lack of confidence was such that she was overcome by her deficiencies as she appreciated their problems.

Since that time I have inclined to believe that students' difficulties in treatment are more likely to arise from lack of confidence than from almost anything else. It is rare that a student suffers from an excess of confidence and needs the salutary effect of a little failure. There are always those, of course, who find it difficult to accept direction and have to find out everything the hard way.

Male students are conspicuous in this respect. Indeed the poor male student in Britain is conspicuous in every respect. In each group he is likely to be unique. One male to seventeen females was the average when I was teaching. Every year we hoped for at least two or three so that ranks could be closed against the monstrous regiment but we invariably ended up with just one.

The reason is a straightforward financial one. Many men are attracted to speech therapy but they cannot afford to practice it in Britain. The salaries are just too low. Unless he has an additional teaching or medical qualification which will increase his earnings and his status the male speech therapist can barely survive here. The majority of those who do qualify, emigrate.

It was a revelation to me to find the field of speech pathology in the United States so dominated by men. It was a considerable surprise to be confronted with a large class of graduate students of which half were men, but it was a very pleasant surprise. It is much more stimulating for everyone to pursue and practice a profession where the sexes are equally divided.

Speech therapy is generally considered to be a woman's profession but I believe this to be a convention relating to the status and earning power of the profession. Men make excellent psycho-therapists and clinical psychologists and are equally adept at speech therapy given the interest and the encouragement. Certainly there is plenty of scope for them in teaching and research into speech disorders.

One of my male students was sent to carry out his clinical observations at a hospital where the therapist was a former fellow student of mine. She reported to me with some amusement that after he had appeared at the clinic several times, sitting firmly and silently in his chair observing her treatment, one of the patients asked what his duties were. On being told that he was a speech therapy student the patient appeared surprised and subsequently confessed that he had believed the male in question to be employed by the hospital to protect the therapist from unseemly advances.

After I had been teaching for some years the need for further study became imperative. I accordingly set about doing some intensive work in a specific area of interest and submitted this, and myself, to the College of Speech Therapists for examination. The work was fascinating and the experience salutary. I had forgotten how difficult it was to be a student and particularly how unpleasant it is to be examined.

I gained my higher qualification and with it a little more insight into the difficult students, whose ranks I considered myself to have joined. These two assets were to be invaluable in my next appointment.

The retirement of the director of the speech therapy department was a notable event in the life of the school, to which she had contributed enormously, and in my own life also because I succeeded her. Both the honour and the responsibility of following this doyenne of speech therapy were certainly felt. Until this time my role had largely been defined by my own behaviour. I was a lecturer and a tutor but my relations with the students could be fairly informal if I wished them to be.

Taking over the directorship of the department necessarily meant an increase in authority both psychological and actual. I surrendered my smaller chores but I inherited bigger ones. Interviewing, marking, letter writing, committees, the hours spent at these all went up and up. Such tasks are important indeed but they can be hard to accept if they rob you too much of time to practise the skill upon which all this edifice has been built.

This is one of the paradoxical features of promotion and not, of course, restricted to speech therapy. One goes into speech therapy because one wants to help people to speak. One becomes sufficiently accomplished at this to start instructing others. Then, imperceptibly, one starts to gather the crust and trappings of the training school teacher. Responsibilities in this area increase, and while they may be enjoyed considerably for what they are, they cannot but take away from what one does best.

It would not be true to say that I resented the loss of clinical time sufficiently to contemplate resigning my appointment and going back into full time clinical work though I might ultimately have done so. To begin with I enjoyed the responsibility and scope of the job enough to compensate for the loss of clinical time. It was satisfying to be able to choose my own staff and select my own students. It was extremely satisfying to have a chance to try out my own ideas.

But it was disconcerting to realise that I had now reached a professional pinnacle. I had inherited one of the top jobs in my profession and might reasonably expect to stay in it for some thirty-five years. I was fortunate, yes, to have this kind of security. But was it the kind of security that I wanted?

I did not have time to become unduly preoccupied with thoughts of my years of tenure, nor my lack of exposure to new experiences. As I pointed out earlier, the development of a therapist is the development of a person. The demands of speechless mankind now had to compete with the demands of one very articulate man. It became important to me that I transfer myself to the United States. It was fortunate for my professional life that the United States was the continent in question. Had it been Antarctica I would certainly have got myself there, but this book would probably now be concluded.

It was extremely hard to leave the Central School which had been part of my life for so many years. It was also hard to leave my patients and my colleagues at the hospital. It is only when a parting is inevitable that the strength of the matrix in which one's life is set becomes fully revealed. But in the Chinese saying 'If you come to a river and you cannot get across, throw your heart across and jump after it'.

It was in this spirit that I crossed the Atlantic.

# 7

# UNITED STATES AND DIFFERING VIEWPOINTS

## *Speech Therapy in America*

FOR THE NEXT FIVE YEARS the site of my personal and professional life was to be a huge university campus in the Mid-West of the United States. A greater contrast to life in London can scarcely be imagined. The cosy compactness of the Central School, London and indeed Britain, was suddenly brought home to me. They had never appeared to possess this attribute while I was actually there and I had spent much time fretting about lack of space on the one hand and diffusion of energies on the other.

Obviously I endowed them in their absence with those aspects that most speak of warmth and familiarity. I find the same distortion creeping in now in attempting to write about America. By the time I left the Mid-West it had become familiar territory. The vast size of the university, at first so unspeakably daunting, now just appears as one of its essential attributes. It is a place where we had a rich and useful life, a place whose organisation I now understand and with whose idiosyncracies I am familiar.

Even the huge territory of the rest of the States has become to me the country where we climbed mountains in the west, where I hunted for shells on Florida beaches, where we held a Cerebral Palsy workshop in Louisiana and followed it by a night out in New Orleans. When I see films or read books set in Chicago or in a small mid-western town, I have immediate memories and associations. I have a way of looking at them which is the result of all the experience the States has yielded me and the personal and professional happiness I found there.

But I cannot pretend that my first days in my new department were spent in anything but amiable directives on the one hand and polite confusion on the other. Everyone attached to it welcomed me with great ease and friendliness, prepared to tell me anything I wanted to know.

Some of my reactions must have been disconcerting to them. For example, why did everyone talk about 'clock hours'? What other kind of hours were there? And the Professor of Audiology who, with kind and charming alacrity, asked me to 'audit' his classes, meaning attend the course without taking an examination, deserved a better response than the disconcerted gape of one to whom audit means 'officially to inspect the books'.

What I needed was someone to explain the whole system to me in simple terms as to a complete outsider, which I was. It took me some time to achieve this because everyone greeted me as a professional colleague, which of course I was also.

At that time it was not possible to study speech therapy at a university in Britain so I was not familiar with a degree course in the subject. Even had I been, it would probably not have helped me because the American system is so different. I had started to perceive some of these differences when I first wrote to find out whether I could work there.

It was by no means easy to get a job in an American university because our diploma did not equate, in American eyes, with their degree. I particularly wanted to work in a university department in order to increase my theoretical knowledge and so it was fortunate for me that this particular department was disposed to consider my higher qualification and teaching experience as evidence that I might be able to do so.

It was still necessary though, for the university administration to accept me. This meant an application giving details of every course taken and subjects studied with all sorts of addenda such as length of courses and numbers of hours spent in supervised reading. This had to be signed by the head of the department and this person being in fact myself made the procedure appear even more ludicrous in my eyes.

But I got it all hammered out onto a nice piece of official notepaper which bore my name as director of the department. I was quite pleased with the result which was really rather impressive. It gained me my appointment and permission to study for a Ph.D., but it was a little disconcerting to come across the whole lot some years later in a folder in the departmental files with scribbled on the outside, 'We think she is worth taking a chance on'.

I hope they still think so. I never did read for a Ph.D. because of my marriage which took place some little time after my arrival in the States. A clinical post was offered to me which seemed to combine much better with marriage and as the clinic was actually held on the university premises there was all the access to books and research findings that one could wish. By that time I was a little more conversant with the system though it was still not crystal clear to me.

Students of speech pathology were required to take certain selected courses as part of their qualification for a degree which had '*practicum*' or practical clinical work. This was necessary at the undergraduate level and also in reading for a Master's degree. This practical work was carried out at clinics organised and supervised by university staff.

Consequently there seemed to be a bewilderment of students all with differing amounts of experience and theoretical knowledge to be absorbed into the clinic and guided through the initiation into its mysteries and demands. Classes in mid-west universities are very large by British standards and it was difficult to remember the name of any student unless he obtruded himself upon your notice in some distinctive manner.

Joe's name was the first I learned and this was because the day after I had met him in clinic I found him serving me in the supermarket. Any service I may have rendered him in the way of clinical elucidation was amply repaid as he guided me through the array of choice, information and temptation with which I was confronted.

There is no doubt that the American system gives the student excellent opportunities for academic study. The theoretical aspects of all subjects pertaining to speech, hearing and language pathology were thoroughly covered in course work. But early in the history of the degree someone had made the quite erroneous assumption that if you give a student a lecture on a certain condition, a number of techniques on how to ameliorate it and a standard textbook to fall back on, he will be able to function as a therapist.

This is just not possible. It is extremely hard for a student to make a transfer from a class lecture to a clinical skill. Information is not enough. Information is contained in the sentence 'the minimally brain damaged child may be hyper-active'. It does not help you when he has climbed from table to wall to window sill and is now tearing up your equipment.

Some treatment appeared easy to teach by rote and articulation therapy was one of them. But faced by the child with an articulation disorder the student needs more than this 'cook book' to fall back on. There are very good 'cook books' in the States that tell you how to obtain success in ninety-nine cases out of a hundred. It is hard on the poor student that his case is invariably the hundredth.

The situation was not made easier for the student by the supervisory arrangements. It used to be common practice for graduates studying for their Ph.D. to supervise students by way of earning money. This could work quite well if the supervisor was an older person with experience of practical work. But sometimes he had just obtained his Master's degree and had had very little more practical experience than the student he was supervising.

The American and British systems seemed to be in direct contrast to each other regarding emphasis. In Britain you were trained as a therapist and taught, by demonstration and by practice, how to treat patients. In the States you were required to study the theory of your subject as an academic discipline and to pursue that study as far as possible.

It is significant that in Britain the student rarely conducted any piece of work that could be called research and equally significant that in the States a mark given for a student's practical work rarely influenced the quality of his degree. British students have been far too limited intellectually and Americans have not all been taught how to become skilful clinicians.

This is now a matter of historical rather than continuing validity. The American Speech and Hearing Association has upgraded its standards for clinical competence and practical work has now been considerably extended and intensified. In Britain we have at last managed to obtain entry into one university and speech therapists are eligible to pursue further study or training in many different educational establishments.

I arrived back in England to find the first degree course established and I left America with my department only employing full-time supervisors with clinical experience. There was also a much more fruitful interchange between clinic and classroom. Professors arranged clinic demonstrations to be given as part of their courses and students were required to start observing in the clinic the year before they were ready for their practicum.

But it was only a short while before I left that I passed a student bustling anxiously down to the clinic to carry out her first voice evaluation with a new patient. It was necessary to respond with an encouraging beam to her brave smile and gently remove from under her arm the text book entitled *Voice Therapy* which might somewhat have reduced the patient's confidence in her ability. I do not doubt that I could have found her prototype in Britain.

A department consisting of clinical, research and teaching personnel is not an easy establishment but if it can be made to work harmoniously it is, of all places, the most stimulating in which to practice one's skill. The rivalries and suspicions between the factions can probably never be entirely dispelled but if kept under control they provide a good edge and keep everyone on their toes.

The clinician can feed the research worker with material and may hope to learn in return what is the rationale on which her treatment is based. She may, of course, work out her rationale for herself in which case it must be firm and sure enough to withstand the questions of those who will only accept statistical evidence. The research worker must contend with the smiles of the clinicians who listen to the painstaking scholarly proof which he has mustered in support of something they find to be clinically self-evident.

Sometimes it seems as though the two aspects of the profession have split too far apart to be able to nourish each other, their language has become too different and their outlook too dissimilar. But given good co-ordination and goodwill the mutual interplay can be extraordinarily rewarding. It is only when the individuals concerned do not really value each other's contribution that the establishment becomes polarised and the students drift between them manipulating and being manipulated.

After so many years in which I had worked as the only speech therapist or the senior or junior in an establishment of two, I never quite got over the sheer pleasure of having so many colleagues to talk to. It was marvellous to be able to march into one of the professors' rooms and say 'What are the present ideas on tongue thrust and what has been written on it in the last few years and is it any good?' and get an answer.

It was a pleasure to stagger into the drug store next door after a long day of diagnostics and know that you would find a group of people who had been involved with you, rubbing their hands or licking their wounds over the day's battles. The drug store became an extension of the department. At any time of day students and staff could be found there in conversation, erudite and otherwise, washed down by draughts of Coke and coffee.

A number of us were there the day that President Kennedy was shot. A student heard the news on his transistor and we all sat, unbelieving and horrified amid the debris of our hamburgers. When we got back to the clinic there was a notice on the bulletin board to say the President was dead.

There was a small boy waiting for his speech and hearing evaluation and we all looked at each other wondering what on earth was the appropriate thing to do. Finally we got on with our work. There seemed no reason to deny him his treatment because of a cataclysm that had barely yet impinged on us. And he had come a long way.

Diagnostics day was the high spot of the week in many ways. On this day children would be brought to the clinic from anywhere in the state and given a full scale speech, hearing and language evaluation. In spite of a certain amount of preparatory information you never really knew what you were getting. Frequently all the family accompanied the silent member and the far from adequate waiting room was strained to its capacity.

There were three supervisors on diagnostics day, the Professor of Audiology, the Professor of Speech Pathology who taught the theory course, and myself. We sorted out our respective patients and students and took up our positions. Each clinic room was equipped with a one-way window and the supervisor would remain behind it for as long as was humanly possible while the student started the investigation.

It was certainly a situation to induce anxiety in everyone; the child wondering what the student was going to do, the supervisor wondering what the child and student were going to do and the student wondering what the child was going to do, what the supervisor was going to do and what on earth she was going to do herself.

It was amazing really that given the circumstances such excellent results were obtained. The tension contributed positively as long as it was kept under control. Everyone was alert and prepared. If people became too nervous of course disintegration set in. Apparatus was dropped, tests were given badly, vital organs

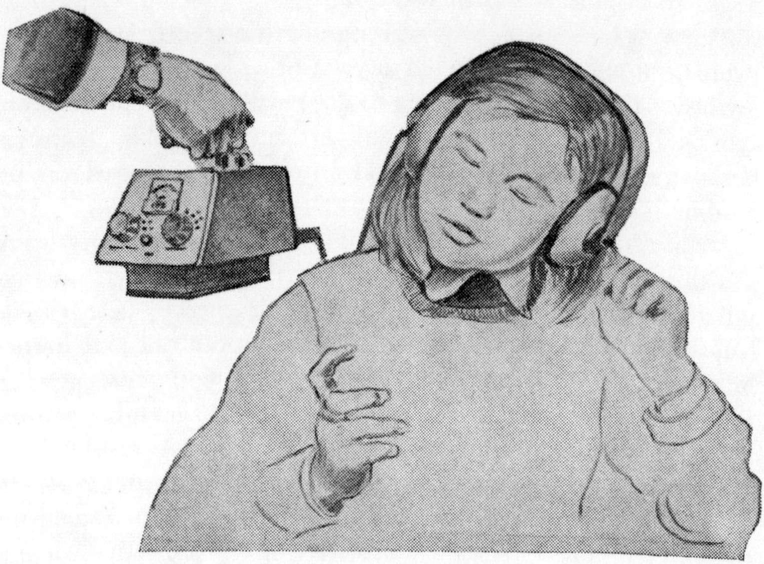

were left uninspected. But if encouraged and supported without too much nagging, a good team of graduate students could often manage a very thorough and useful evaluation.

Sometimes if things were going well one could leave one's post and look to see what kind of child the others had drawn.

I particularly liked to watch my colleagues testing because each had a clinical expertise which was a pleasure to see. The extent and kind of the hearing testing was much less familiar to me then than it is now. Hearing loss is one thing that must not be overlooked in a young child.

Early speech and language teaching is vital if the child is to learn to communicate and the longer he goes without such training the more linguistically retarded he will be. A young child who has come a long way and is apprehensive and irritable is a difficult subject for assessment. But rarely was a child sent away without the tests being completed. It was beautiful to see the dynamic, patient and reassuring interaction which gradually revealed the clinical picture.

Frequently we carried out diagnostic evaluations for demonstration purposes. At the end of the semester we would conduct a diagnostic examination. Students would observe all the procedures and then make up their own minds as to the condition. It was important, of course, not to choose children who were severely deaf or had some outstanding defect that made them diagnostically easy.

But this was no problem. There never seemed to be any dearth of complicated little children waiting for speech assessments. And if there had been I do not doubt that the course instructor would have whipped up some alternative.

Years of teaching diagnostics combined with a capacity for work which surpassed that of Hercules and a devotion to the cause which exceeded Joan of Arc's, meant that this resourceful woman was never at a loss. Starting her classes at seven-forty-five and working straight through a day of therapy, teaching, meetings and interviews, she was still able to give out a little extra energy to support a decadent British colleague who had only started work at nine.

It is apparently my lot in life to be shamed and stimulated by the extraordinary energy and devotion of my female colleagues.

'If you want anything done', I would mutter as this one dashed off a few reports, reorganised the diagnostic timetable, collected us all coffee from the drug store and interviewed a few students for reassurance or reprimand, 'If you want anything done, give it to a busy person'.

# 8

## SUMMER SCHOOL WITH THE SPEECH DISORDERED

### *Residential Speech Therapy*

WHEN I LEFT ENGLAND I carried with me the results of my training and experience but I left behind the social, medical and educational setting within which they had operated.

Had I pursued a course of academic study in the States the absence of this environment would not have struck me so forcibly. I would have been predominantly concerned for some years with the university environment and would have been in some measure protected from the need to explore outside. But with the decision to spend the main part of my time in clinical work came the responsibility to find out much more about the setting in which rehabilitation and re-education could operate.

Working in Britain in so many different areas, both geographical and professional, meant that I had absorbed what I needed to know about the society in which my patients were attempting to function by a process of osmosis rather than concentrated learning. Sometimes of course, the change in law, rearrangement of authority and regrouping of districts meant that a spell of concentrated application had to be put in. But on the whole it was a gradual extension of knowledge learnt in a practical working situation and therefore retained without difficulty.

Given a speech handicapped child or adult I knew the demands of his particular social or educational environment, I knew the medical services which were open to him and who could assist him to obtain them. I was also thoroughly familiar with the organisation of my profession so that, while it might frustrate, it no longer bewildered.

The manner in which to prepare students for College examination, the way in which these examinations were carried out and the significance of the results, these were now a matter of immediate recognition. I had sat on the Council of the College of Speech Therapists and worked on its committees, thus becoming conversant with its ways and helping to shape its policy. In so far as anyone can be said to know their professional environment, I knew mine.

This was all stripped away when I changed countries. Consequently the help that I could give an individual or a community was accordingly reduced. There are many educational and medical specialities where knowledge can be transferred *in toto* from one community to another. I do not believe this to be true of speech therapy. The kind of communication a person needs depends very much on the community within which he functions.

Obviously in all the major ways society in the States and England is very similar. The same motivations and constraints operate. But even apparently small variations can make a considerable difference to the emphasis that is placed on speech. For example, children in Britain start compulsory schooling at five, in the States at six. In Britain there is consequently more pressure from parents and teachers to clear up any minor articulatory problems at a slightly earlier age than in the States in order not to interfere with reading.

I had expected that the English child might be under more pressure to improve his speech because of the dominance of the social class system. While emphasis on Received Pronunciation or Standard English has declined and regional accents are almost *de rigueur*, there is still a solid middle class block which expects a child to demonstrate his social advantages by speaking intelligibly and with pleasing effect at an early age.

But I found that the pressure upon the young child in the Mid-West community where I worked was certainly as great. Social distinctions did not need to be revealed by clear, pleasant speech but superior intelligence must be revealed as soon as possible by superior fluency. Consequently one found all the signs of parental anxiety and mismanagement in one country as in another.

One also encountered individual cases which could have been reproduced, and indeed were reproduced, on each side of the Atlantic. I can recall two adolescent spastic girls, one from a small Mid-Western village, the other from a London suburb, both telling me how acutely they felt their lack of ability to enter into the teenage world with its over-riding emphasis on 'dates' or 'boy friends'. I remember talking to the wife of an elderly aphasic patient in the States and hearing of his social isolation.

'No-one seems to want to drop in for a cup of coffee and a chat. I know it's difficult for them as he can't speak back but it would be company for us'. I returned to hear almost the same words from a wife in the north of England.

'We hoped that people would come and see us as it's difficult for us to move about. But they don't do it. I think that they are embarrassed because he can't talk to them. But if they only knew what a difference it would make to him'.

In my London hospital I had left a woman who had had severe vocal difficulties starting from the death of her parents and the consequent need to take over their business. In the States I found her double, another conscientious over-worked spinster trying too hard to accept a way of life that was both over-demanding and unsatisfactory and whose conflicts were reflected in her vocal strain.

People and problems may be the same but conditions by which they can be resolved alter. An outstanding difference between the two countries was, of course, the presence or absence of the National Health Service. I had worked within this service for years and automatically assumed that if a child needed a hearing aid, an operation for a cleft palate or speech therapy, he could have it. The possibility of its being refused him because the family could not afford to pay for it simply did not occur to me.

Our clinic was subsidised by the University as it operated for teaching and research purposes and so no child was refused treatment even if the family could not pay. But this gave a considerable number of headaches to the administration. We were not really a service clinic and our staff was meant to be developing new skills and techniques in special conditions, not working themselves so hard in providing routine treatments that there was no time or energy left for teaching or research.

It was obviously necessary and important that good co-operative arrangements were worked out between all the speech and hearing services in the area. Consequently the university woıked very closely with the department responsible for the services throughout the state and the school authorities responsible for them in the city.

My first intensive working contact with the members of the State department came with my first summer clinic. American schools and universities have a very long summer break as their working year is divided into two semesters instead of three terms. As speech therapists in the school service have school holidays, children would have an excessively long interruption to their treatment unless special arrangements were made.

Students too, would probably not be able to reach degree level at the required time without the extra points collected by attending 'summer school'. So a joint clinic was run by State and university in which children were brought in from all over the State and boarded out in the town. They would then be brought in to a building specially taken over for the purpose and given intensive speech therapy daily by students supervised jointly by university personnel and speech therapists from the State.

It was a remarkable project in its demands on planning and

organisation, care and co-operation. It meant that children from isolated rural areas who might otherwise not get speech therapy at all could be treated and their difficulties explained to the school staff together with all possible recommendations for help.

It meant that the students received an opportunity to get to know the children and to achieve something in treatment to a much greater extent than could be provided by any other method. But for the supervisors it was eight weeks of operating on the edge of chaos, eight weeks of sheer, concentrated hard labour.

So I cannot understand why, having barely survived the first summer and emerged emotionally exhausted and physically reduced, I should have eagerly and enthusiastically volunteered for a second. And this I did, not with the suicidal blindness of the lemming or the stoicism of a Sidney Carton, but with positive convinced, volition. I can only think it was the children.

When I first requested an opportunity to work in the university clinic I had referred to my interest in language problems in children and my wish to study them more closely. This had not been forgotten and the group that fell to my lot was the language disordered. This consisted of children between the ages of eight and eleven who were attending normal school but who were showing all kinds of learning and frequently behaviour problems which seemed to stem from their disordered and confused speech.

The number was meant to be kept down to sixteen or so, but it invariably sneaked up to eighteen. As the criteria for selection was the child's need, the homogeneity of the group was not a first factor. In fact, it never became a factor at all.

Each child formed, in the words of a past President of the Speech and Hearing Association, a class of one. And thus each child, in the setting of that summer school with its daily programme, its humour, desperation and temperatures of ninety-five degrees, is indelibly imprinted upon my memory.

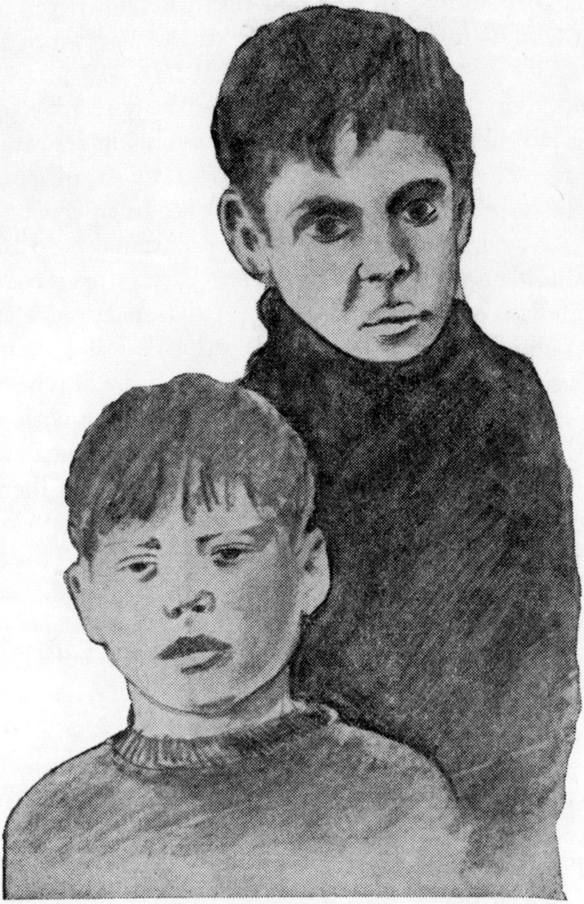

The one thing the children had in common, apart from their disordered speech and language, was an obvious and pervasive feeling of failure. These children had, for years, been bottom of the class in almost every subject, for there are few subjects that do not require a basic level of competence in language.

Their spelling was usually wildly different from the conventional versions and frequently their poor ability to learn by ear made them seem deliberately inattentive to instruction and teaching. So they all had a hang-dog look or a belligerent look. Most of them also had poor physical co-ordination so they no more shone in games than they did in study.

Now, in a group of children with similar difficulties, everyone could be a success. Indeed, it was a major part of the therapy to see that everyone was. Competition was kept to a minimum because if somebody won somebody else had to lose and these children had been losers for too long. There was a general atmosphere of relaxation, ease, encouragement and understanding to which the students contributed very well, allaying their own anxieties when faced with the children's.

There was also a firm and well controlled timetable and a few basic rules strongly reinforced. This was necessary to prevent complete chaos because these children were less able to organise themselves than the average child and, without a certain amount of structure, activities would end in disaster.

It was no easy thing to devise a programme for these children that would keep them stimulated and happy without overloading them. They had to work hard to make progress but if pushed too far they would naturally become rebellious. Speech therapy was given in large groups, small groups and individually, each student being responsible for two children.

Work was done on language and vocabulary building, production of sounds and words that caused particular difficulty, ear training and co-ordination. These activities were carried out individually. In groups we tried to find ways of applying the new learning to games. Sometimes the children acted plays or sang to us. And sometimes we reciprocated. Most of the children settled in well and enjoyed the activities. Some did not.

The child I remember as holding out longest was Gerry, an extremely intelligent boy with unintelligible speech. He had now got his family well organised to understand his gesture and if they did not understand what he was asking for, he took it anyway. At school he was a conspicuous 'loner' and the teacher was divided between real feeling for the boy's difficulties and exasperation at his refusal to co-operate. He was apparently capable of refusing to do something more often and sticking to his refusal longer than any child previously known to her and after a day in his company I could believe it.

I have often remarked to the students that children have few weapons, but the ones they have are extremely effective. They can cry, they can fight, they can become quite silent, they can be sick. Gerry did them all. The first time he felt sick he was given the benefit of the doubt and allowed to go back to his housemother who reported that he had perked up and been as chirpy as a cricket all day.

The second time he appeared with a worried student and a limp look I was prepared. I was ready to allow him to sit quietly in a corner but he had to stay. Gerry's graphic gestures informed me what might be the consequences of his detention. I remained adamant. I would like to report that I won that round but alas, Gerry recovered his health only to demonstrate his ability to crawl under a large pile of desks and remain there for longer than would have been thought possible.

This kind of behaviour obviously has to be dealt with effectively because, if not, all the children become infected. It is very hard on the students also. I went down to talk to the psychologist who had a nice quiet room at the end of the corridor where children could be given intelligence tests or helpful talks. Gerry, I was informed, had a high degree of anxiety. So, I responded, had I. Was it going to help the child to be permissive with him or should we fight back?

On the whole the psychologist thought that so long as we did not push the child too far we should place demands on him. We both felt that this behaviour was an attempt to protect himself from direct speech work. Gerry was much too intelligent to want to move in to an area where he did not expect to have success. By far the most helpful thing we could do would be to make some progress with him towards intelligibility.

Thus supported we moved in. My colleague and I took over the speech work to begin with and made it quite clear that a certain amount of effort on his part would result in privileges, but no attempt meant not much fun either. This would not have worked had we not been able to help him achieve success. But by presenting him with a series of simple sounds to work on until he became more confident and then gradually inserting harder ones, we were genuinely able to praise him and reward his progress. He in turn applied his wits to going one better and started to surprise us by his own variations on the sounds we taught him.

It was terribly hard to see him go at the end of the eight week session knowing that we had only just started to get somewhere.

At the end of each morning a member of staff demonstrated treatment methods for the benefit of the students. One boy, Chris, had an extraordinarily recalcitrant tongue and so one day I used a contrast stimulation technique to get some movement going which involved alternatively scratching it with a wooden tongue blade and then applying a piece of ice to the tip.

With the temperature now at ninety-six and no air conditioning, this became the most popular treatment in the building and I had to discourage it before the kitchen staff became too vociferous over their lost ice and the children started asking for it in assorted flavours!

The parents of every child visited us at least once during his stay and frequently his class teacher or speech therapist would come also. These visits were essential and usually highly productive. It is simply no use for a number of specialists to work with children unless their findings can be shared by the people who see the child every day. It was necessary to explain what the difficulties were and how they might best be tackled. Sometimes this meant direct help with speech, sometimes the much less tangible but vital areas of general handling.

When the children left we had to set to to write the most full and helpful reports we could and these, together with the psychologists' findings, were sent to the state department for information and so that the work might be supplemented. The state supervisors would then visit the children as often as possible to follow up the suggestions made.

Ours was not the only group to receive such attention. There was also a group for the young hard-of-hearing child, another for adolescent stammerers and a nursery type group for the very young cleft palates. Each group received the same level of attention and care, initial assessments, treatment and then follow up visits. The whole project must have taken a very high degree of planning.

My involvement in its showed me something of the work that has to be done by conscientious officers who carry responsibility for the welfare of the handicapped and it left me full of admiration for their activities. People who organise such projects seem to me to have so many headaches and so few rewards compared to those of us that actually work with the children.

We may hope to see a change of attitude, a newly acquired consonant, a more easily produced sentence almost every day. We have the fun of their communications and the warmth of their affection. And for these rewards the extra grey hair, the occasional headache, the frequent exhaustion and the slightly frayed temper seems a small price to pay.

# 9

## 'GEE, IT MUST BE TOUGH ON YOU'

### *Speech Therapy for Aphasic and Autistic Children*

An immediate and predictable result of working with the language disordered children of eight and above was the determination to seek out similar children at a much younger age and start working with them before constriction had become clamped upon confusion and while there was a good chance of helping them to acquire basic knowledge about language in a more systematic way.

This wish to work with very young children had been strong in me before I left England. Many of us felt increasingly that, as so many speech defects and disorders stemmed from inability to appreciate some of the important sound distinctions in a language, we should try to stimulate the young child to listen before his ability to do so declined further. It also seemed very important to help the mother, in particular, to handle the young child appropriately during the vital time for language growth.

When speech is delayed parents become worried and this anxiety is, of course, communicated unconsciously to the child. When he does finally reach a milestone in speech, his first word or his first sentence, the reception may not so much be spontaneous pleasure by the parents but 'Thank goodness he's done it at last'. Which is not nearly so encouraging.

This kind of response by parents is very common among those with mentally retarded children. While it is not at all true to say that all children with language difficulties are mentally retarded, it is probably true to say that all mentally retarded children have language difficulties. What is now emerging is the fact that they are often retarded still further by their language limitations and so do not function in any intellectual area as well as they might do because of this.

Another group that might well have basic language problems is the emotionally disturbed, containing among others, the autistic child. These children's outstanding inability is in the whole field of communication, so impaired capacity to cope with spoken language could be a contributory factor.

I think every therapist will remember her first experience of meeting an autistic child. Mine was with a little coloured boy who was attending a day centre in London to which I was taken by a child psychiatrist. This child was playing with a humming top, pushing the plunger up and down to make it work and gently crooning to himself as he did so. When we spoke to him he did not respond, his eyes never focused upon us and he turned immediately from our touch.

Watching him one felt completely extraneous, an object unable to impinge upon the boy's attention. Another child stole the top and playing with it clumsily, broke it. The teacher, the psychiatrist and I all tried to mend it but unsuccessfully. So we laid it aside and continued our discussion. After a while the humming noise started up again and we saw the little coloured boy, having completed his repair, playing once more with his toy with the same complete absorption as before.

There was another group of language disturbed children which was also of outstanding interest. These were the children who were unable to understand or produce language because their ability to handle its symbolic structure had not developed. When we use the word 'table' we are in fact producing a speech symbol for the actual object. We do not need to see a table in front of us to make it clear to other people. The word will do.

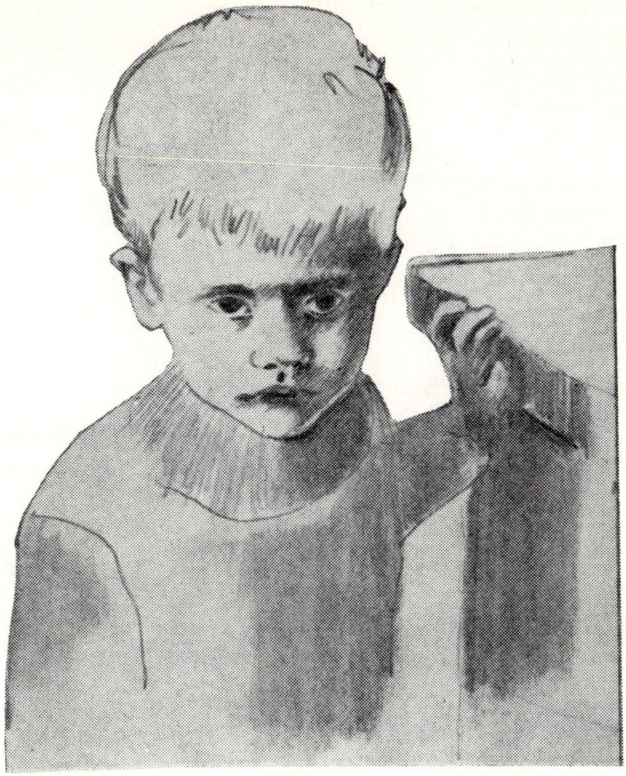

This sort of behaviour is, of course, only possible if the whole community agrees on the symbols it is to use. But for most of us this is not a matter of choice. We hear the spoken word at the same time as we first see the object, we accept that this is the name for this particular thing.

Some children are just not able to do this. They cannot associate the spoken word with the object, they cannot remember it or they cannot reproduce it. They will be quite unable to communicate unless taught by special means. At first they may be thought to be deaf because of their lack of interest in speech and it is very important for their future welfare and for their education that they are diagnosed as early as possible.

When I was a student the first school for these children had been opened in England. But it could take very few out of the number needing help. Hope for the future probably lay in early diagnosis and pre-school work which might help the less severe to cope in normal classrooms and so leave such schools to deal with the children who were so handicapped that they could not respond in any way to ordinary teaching.

So all of us who saw the difficulties of the school-aged child, struggling with inadequate language to establish himself in a world dominated by language, felt a tremendous responsibility to identify similar difficulties as soon as possible so that the child might be helped as much, and distressed as little, as could be.

I had seen all these children in my school and hospital clinics where treatment for them can be frustrating because it is usually so inadequate. Twice-weekly therapy is quite insufficient to explore the problem let alone find the solution and in many instances the child was not even able to receive that. I felt that if I knew a little more, or rather a greal deal more, about language disorders, I could put my treatment time to much better effect by using it for demonstration to parents who could then carry out more work at home.

The United States was the ideal place to learn more about diagnosis and treatment. Its immense resources meant that it could provide superbly equipped premises—diagnostic and treatment centres and schools for every kind of communication handicap. The study of the underlying conditions at university level meant that money was usually available through education grants. Consequently teams of experts could be gathered together to operate research and treatment programmes. Audiologists, psychologists and speech therapists could be housed together in one department so that interaction and exchange of information was a matter of daily occurrence.

I do not wish to imply that the United States is one hundred per cent enlightened and that Britain is, in these matters, a backward country. I have never felt this to be true. Britain contains individual neurologists, psychologists, audiologists and speech therapists whose care and clinical expertise is as great as can be found anywhere in the world. But we do lack training facilities and this is a matter of economic priorities. There are many of us learning on the job who would gain immeasurably from time off to observe and study under the guidance of experienced people.

For my part I think much of what I saw in the States would have been wasted on me without the learning on the job which had preceded it. I would have been overwhelmed by the abundance of everything and unable to isolate the important things. I might have been too easily impressed on the one hand and unable to appreciate significant factors on the other. I was, I believe, ideally placed for benefitting from what was offered to me because of all the failure and success, exposure and limitations that I had encountered as a therapist.

But I could not have hoped to be given so much, and so generously. This was a bonus indeed. Had my marriage taken me to another part of the States I might perhaps have been equally fortunate. But it is difficult to believe. We all know the saying 'Never the time, the place and the loved one', but not all of us are fortunate enough to be able to disprove it.

The department in which I worked already comprised professors and courses in Speech Pathology, Audiology and Voice Science. During the time I was there it also established degree work in Language. A new professor was appointed to organise the courses and to teach the theory. This meant that it was now possible for me to attend seminars and lectures upon aspects of language which I would otherwise never have been exposed to.

We were also able to set up experimental programmes with all the groups of children which I have just described. So one of the things I particularly wished to do was made possible for me. So was the other but it proved to be unrealistic. It was the wish I had expressed to learn to evaluate, objectively, the results of my therapy. This is something we all want to do. When a method works we want to know why it works and the likelihood of its working again. We want to know whether our therapy has made any difference and if so what were the crucial factors that really made the difference.

Such questions have often been raised about medicine. Is it the drug or what Dr. Michael Balint called 'dose doctor' that produces the improvements? They have also been raised about teaching. To what extent is any new teaching method successful because of the enthusiasm of the teachers who promote it and to what extent to its intrinsic value?

So with speech therapy. We feel we need objective criteria to establish ourselves, in our own minds and those of other people, as useful professional workers. I have pointed out before that it is easy to become discouraged about therapy. If the child improves it is maturation and if he does not it is your fault.

I now doubt that such objective criteria are ever going to be possible. In fact I no longer feel at all strongly about the need for them. The important thing is that progress takes place and we are all as honest as possible about our own contributions. Authorities are certainly convinced by control group studies but it is my experience that they are also convinced by human need. We are now sent many severely handicapped children for therapy in order that parents may be prevailed upon to accept them with less distress and the family can consequently live more fully.

The kind of advice and support one gives in these situations is not directly measurable in terms of words learned or sounds uttered. But it is very important that false hopes are not raised and time and money are not wasted by the continuance of a therapy programme from which little benefit is derived by anyone in proportion to the effort expended.

The language programme established under the new course certainly made an effort to produce objective criteria but, by the time I left, things were still very much in the preliminary stages. It is extremely difficult to control all the necessary factors in this kind of research. There are just too many of them. I later assisted on a project organised by one of the state psychologists to assess improvement in school children under different classroom conditions. My little area just concerned speech and language and even that was difficult enough to consider. I have amused and affectionate memories of the poor man wandering into my room saying, 'It started as a nice clean piece of research and it's just getting dirtier and dirtier'.

But even if one cannot establish with objective proof the value of a therapy method it is highly beneficial to have to take a good, long, hard look at it. The language programme was excellent here because we were all able to take some good, long, hard looks at ourselves and each other.

Our centres for treatment were set up in a school for the educationally sub-normal, an institution for the severely retarded and an institution for the emotionally disturbed. We also ran a daily nursery type programme for young children with severely delayed or deviate language. I felt particularly excited about this last group with its possibilities of forestalling some of the severe conditions that proved so intractable. And it was a lovely project. The children were so individual and so appealing, and of course, we got to know them so well.

We tried to give the children a variety of simple experiences to which we could link speech and language. This reproduced the situation which naturally takes place when a mother talks to her child. Only here it was taking place a year or two later and with a little extra reinforcement.

'Ba'.

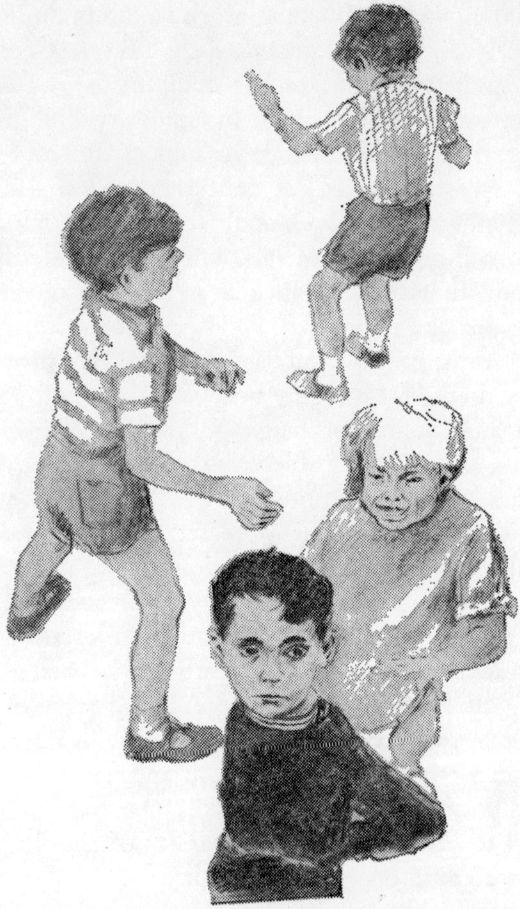

'Here's the ball Jimmy. Do you want to catch it?'

'No, me'.

'All right, (or rather Okay), you throw it'.

'Gone'.

'No, here it is'.

'More frow'.

'Yes, throw it again'.

Our group activities might involve playing at shopping, cooking, taking imaginary trips and sometimes actual ones to the farm, the zoo, the supermarket and the fire station. This last visit was organised by one of my colleagues and it seemed a courageous venture though one fraught with hazard. But it was a great success.

First, one of the firemen visited us and showed us his helmet and his special coat. The children were allowed to try them on while we took advantage of their interest to try to teach them words like 'hot' and 'heavy'. Then the actual visit took place and the children had the great good fortune to be there when a fire warning was given and the men came sliding down the pole in response to the siren.

Play for some time after that was dominated by the fighting of imaginary fires, shouts for 'water' and siren noises. The siren is a satisfying sound for children to imitate as I had previously discovered at the regular clinic. The mother of a pair of particularly energetic and inarticulate twins had driven in from the small village where they lived with reports of the family's increasing unpopularity.

'There's no other kids that can imitate the siren like those two can. They've had the whole village out three times already and what will happen if they do it again, I just don't know'.

It isn't the visits to the fire station or the games of ball which are important. It is the manner in which speech can be linked to the activities so that the children realise that things have a name, that by uttering a certain sound you can make things happen.

The first time a child really makes a connection between the sound he utters and the way someone responds is a tremendously exciting and important moment. We were to see this happen with many of our children and it never lost its thrill. For me though the most vivid recollection of such an occurrence is of an incident that took place in London.

I was working at the hospital with a little girl of five who had no speech and very limited ability to understand language. She came from a very poor home where the mother had severe psychological problems which had meant that the child's handicap escaped notice until she started school. Once there she was immediately shipped off to the hospital for diagnosis and treatment but it was heart breakingly late to be starting with her. It was also difficult to get through to her by other means than gesture.

One day we were both a little exhausted by the effort to make and maintain connection so I walked her down to the hospital shop. It seemed likely that the word 'sweet' might impinge, as food is a great motivator. We had bought our sweets (which I was later forced to call 'candy') and were returning down the corridor when we passed a pram containing a baby of about ten months. Everyone loves a baby so we stopped and indulged in a little cooing.

As we moved off I said to Yvonne, 'Say bye bye'. After I had repeated a few times 'bye bye' and 'bye bye baby' to Yvonne she got the idea. She turned back to the baby and pronounced 'bye bye'.

The baby, who had previously not impressed me by his intelligence and who had made no response to my words of farewell, now showed himself to be a really perceptive and useful child. As Yvonne uttered the magic sounds he lifted a limp little hand and flapped it twice in a gesture of farewell. Yvonne was confounded with delight and astonishment at the effect of her words and could have remained there all the afternoon stimulating the required response if I had not become afraid that the baby would cease to be so obliging and dragged Yvonne away while the lesson was still clear.

We had to work at this level of simple stimulus and response with the very retarded children in our programme. They were at a stage of development where only very simple sound combinations and words could be expected but it was very important that their understanding and use of words should be increased. Children in an institution have been shown to be retarded in their speech, even if they are intelligent, because of the lack of individual attention compared with the child in the home. If they are not intelligent it is even more difficult for them to be motivated to talk.

One reason is, of course, the lack of time the staff can spend with each child but another is certainly the difficulty most people experience in speaking naturally to people who cannot talk back. I have mentioned this in connection with the adult aphasic but it is also true of deafness and cerebral palsy. So the child's environment becomes more and more silent and it is less and less easy for him to make the effort, which for him is an effort, to communicate by speech.

Repetition is basic in helping retarded children to learn words. They must hear the word a number of times and at moments when their attention is held by the object or activity the word represents. And then it must be worth their while to say the word themselves. Something must happen. It is hard to arrange for all this in an institution where there are few staff and hundreds of children.

I was lecturing once to a conference of workers in the field of mental retardation and had spent some time on the necessity to repeat a word, reward the child's attempt and then repeat the word again for him. At question time the first person to rise said, 'I am the only therapist for five hundred severely retarded children'.

But one must preach counsels of perfection even if one has to compromise. These children need to be talked to. And they must try to talk back. We who are competent in language can say a name after hearing it once, can pronounce a word after one demonstration and can make a statement about a completely new experience. These children are quite unable to do this. The gap between our competence and their limitations can only be brought together by simple repetition in pleasant situations. I remember being freshly confounded by this discrepancy when I dropped in to visit a little group of retarded adults who were working together with a teacher in the institution. They were learning their names.

'Good morning Mike. Good morning Sylvia. Good morning Bernard. Good morning Allen. Good morning Joan. Joan, say good morning to Mike, Mike, say good morning to Sylvia. Sylvia, say good morning to Bernard', and so on. The teacher must have spent a good five minutes on this procedure, patiently and clearly saying each pupil's name over and over again. Then, turning to me.

'Won't you come and say Hallo to us?' Up I went.

'Hello Mike. Hello Sylvia. Hello Bernard. Hello Allen. Hello Joan'.

'Why,' remarked the teacher, 'she knows all our names'.

In the educationally sub-normal school most of the children had developed language to some extent and could frequently converse quite well. Our job there was to help them to be intelligible to outside people. A slightly retarded person who can speak clearly and attend to the speech of others is a much better proposition from the point of view of employment than is a person with the same level of intelligence who cannot express himself and is not at ease in communicating with others.

So a certain amount of our work was directed towards speech that would be useful in future employment. I remember one student having a really good time with an adolescent girl who was very good at sewing. When I went in the table was covered with scraps of material whose relative merits were being discussed, increasing vocabulary in the one and a new interest in the other.

The toughest children to work with were the emotionally disturbed. This was due to their unpredictable behaviour and lack of interest in communication but also, of course, to the lack of affection they showed. These are children who have learned, or have been born knowing, not to trust people. They don't smile at you when you go in nor take your hand, nor wave goodbye. At least, not at first.

Their first response to you as a person is something you do not forget. One little girl of six gave me a perfectly horrible time one day, refusing to sit down, throwing things, spitting, running away. After twenty minutes I had had enough. I literally did not know what to do next. It was then she spoke her first word to me. 'Hi', she said anxiously, peering into my face for a response from me. 'Hi'.

Another disturbed child we worked with was living at home and attending a day centre. Her mother used to talk to me a good deal and one day she said, 'You know it really is something that the girls here will work with our kids. We know how beastly they can be. It is hard to keep trying to do something for someone that never seems to love you back. We're stuck with them and it's not so hard for us to love them. But gee, it must be tough on you'.

That woman had to cope all the time with a rebellious, disturbed adolescent who shut herself in her room, threw her food off the table, refused to wash and who had not spoken to her mother all week to punish her for spending a day visiting friends. I looked through the window at the girl who was working quite amiably with a student. She was a nice looking girl and we would soon be handing her back to her mother while we went off to relax with our friends and families.

'It's not hard' I thought, 'for us to love them. But gee, it must be tough on you'.

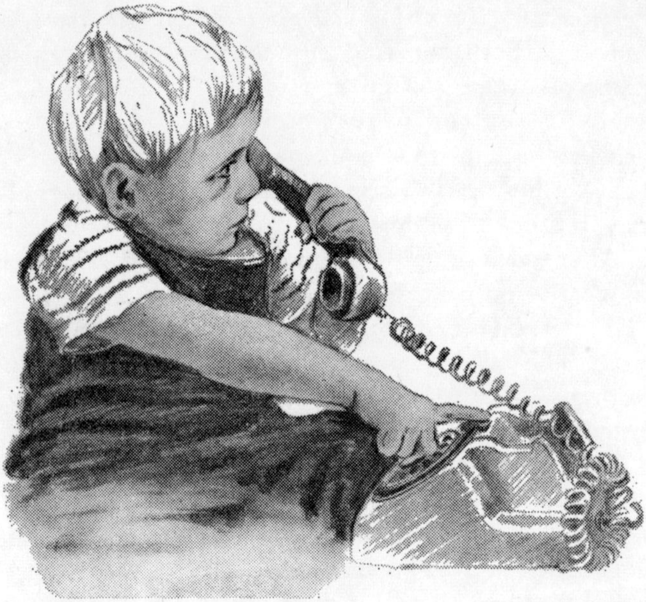

# 10

## COMMUNICATIONS, CONFERENCES, DEMONSTRATIONS AND DISASTERS

No description of a speech therapist's career would be complete without some reference to the conferences, congresses or conventions which one attends. Speech therapy impinges upon so many other subjects that the number of such assemblies open to us is quite considerable. We may find papers to interest us, and perhaps an audience to listen to us, at gatherings of audiologists, linguists and phoneticians, and at congresses medical, psychological and educational. In addition there are our own particular speech therapy conferences where, protected from outside attack, we may challenge each other's ideas with vigour and candour.

In Britain the national speech therapy conferences are comparatively small affairs but in the United States they are enormous. This is not just because of the relative size of each nation but because in the States they have very sensibly and logically refused to have an arbitrary division between speech and hearing pathology and treatment. Consequently the major association is the Association of Speech and Hearing and its numbers are very great. Its annual conventions are held in some important and accessible city, several hotels being taken over for the purpose.

Anyone who has been to one of these conventions will immediately recall the throngs of highly vocal people waiting to register and subsequently to invade all the principal lecture rooms, material exhibitions and, of course, bars that are offered. I was quite overwhelmed on the first occasion and scarcely less on the second and spent much anxious time clutching and studying my programme of events and trying to locate the rooms in which these events were to take place.

The A.S.H.A. also covered the area of Voice Science which would, in this country, tend to come under Phonetics or Physiology. This section enlarged the programme but for many of us was too specialised to enlarge the choice of papers to attend. And this was just as well. The choice was wide enough. Simultaneous papers were presented on many different aspects of speech, hearing and language pathology and therapy and it behoved you to study your programme and place your bets on the likely winners well in advance.

Two main types of convention members could be identified. The older habitués would study their programmes well before arrival, select a few papers in their areas of interest or competence and visit these. They would contribute to the discussion of the papers and then repair to the coffee lounge or bar to pursue annually initiated conversations with colleagues or to recruit new members for their staff. They would return to their departments saying that there were far too many delegates and the quality of the papers was disappointing but it was worth going because of the people who were there.

The less mature, more eager or more suggestible convention members would rush frantically from room to room and paper to paper always in pursuit of the next speaker and always missing the only contribution considered to be important. As all the rooms would be full when they arrived they were forced to stand in the crowded and inaudible areas at the back and never took part in the discussion because they were too afraid of missing what was being said next door.

They would buttonhole people at every meal and party and repair to the bar in any spare minute to counteract the ravages of exhaustion. They too would return to their departments saying that there were far too many delegates and the quality of the papers was disappointing but it was worth going because of the people who were there.

I certainly found the people there of very great interest and was fascinated to meet and talk with those giants who had previously been names on text books or research articles. Another enjoyable aspect was the freedom from any kind of organisational responsibility, a situation all too rare in England.

I was working in London when we had our first meeting in this country of the International Association of Logopaedics and Phoniatrics. My services as a helper were volunteered by the head of my department who was the president of the Association at that time. It was an honour that I shared with many young speech therapists in the home counties, indeed all those who were not quick-witted enough to find excuses in time, nor slow witted enough to be a positive liability. It was impressed upon us all that the success of such a conference is dependent upon the attention to detail by all members of the conference staff and unobtrusive efficiency was to be our watchword.

At the first meeting I volunteered for registration and timing duties with a quickness that I learned from Youth Hostelling where one shouts for 'Sweeping' knowing that potato peeling will be coming up. Registration is always rather alarming because of the large number of foreign visitors that arrive at the same time, but are otherwise unconnected and want to change their currency, the titles of their papers and their hotel accommodation simultaneously.

But it is well worth doing because you meet and identify people right at the beginning of the conference instead of finding too late that the person who was behind you in the coffee queue was the one person you wanted to speak to but he was not wearing his identification tag and you thought he was one of the caterers. I was reasonably successful with my registering if the criteria were the number of people admitted to the conference and the number of times I was invited out subsequently. I was less successful with my timing job, or rather, paradoxically, I was far too successful with it.

Our organisers had impressed upon us the necessity of keeping the participants strictly to their allotted time and not allowing them to stray over into the next speaker's allocation. This is always a problem at a large conference. It is necessary to limit speakers and everyone knows this but most people hope that they will be the one exception that is really welcome. Flashing lights had proved to be unsuccessful in stopping such determined performers and we were given buzzers with instructions to buzz once briefly, a second time more lengthily and finally continuously until the stage was yielded.

It all sounded rather rude but the speakers were warned and were pretty amicable about it. The person who really outwitted us was an American professor who showed a film of himself conducting therapy and talked all the way through it at breakneck speed raising his voice to shout himself down.

I was a little upset to see that my first victim was a very eminent and austere physician, a renowned authority whose pronouncements I was accustomed to receiving with bated breath. On this occasion my breath was bated throughout his delivery and I became more and more uncomfortable as the limit approached. The time came, and passed, and he was still in full exposition with no peroration or prayer in sight.

I stuck it out until my fear of retribution from the organisers became greater than my fear of retribution from the gods and then advanced my finger towards the buzzer. As he paused after a carefully weighed sentence I gave him a wee buzz. He immediately threw down his paper, walked straight off the platform and out of the conference hall, not to return. I sat transfixed by the responsibility of my action glaring miserably at the little buzzer which had robbed the eager swine of so many pearls.

I remember this conference with great affection because it was held in Westminster during a period of such lovely weather that the river and buildings stood out against the golden light as in a Canaletto and we could take our visitors by boat all the way to Greenwich in full pride of place and sunshine and not a mackintosh in sight. We held evening parties in the gardens of all the wealthiest and most horticulturally gifted members of the committee and suddenly our professional life became something of glamour and excitement, with an episodic charm one only thinks to find on holiday, not in the excursions of one's daily job.

The first time I read a paper at a conference was also in London. This was a national conference organised by the College of Speech Therapists and its theme was the Seven Ages of Man. The speech disorder and other communication problems of all the different ages were presented from the infant 'mewling and pewking' to the 'lean and slippered pantaloon' who fell to my lot. I had some experience of the geriatric patient and together with a colleague set out to describe some of the communication difficulties of old age and the role of the speech therapist in ameliorating them. I have always been very grateful for this opportunity. As so often happens, the necessity to clarify and organise one's work for presentation to others gives it a sharpened focus which deepens one's own interest.

The speech disabilities of old age add so much to the patient's dependency and feeling of humiliation and it is important indeed that we should look at these, not just with sympathy but with practical resource. Had I not had to make this particular study my own therapy might have been much less thorough and probably less hopeful than it subsequently became.

From then on I was convinced that to take part in conferences is not just the act of the determined public speaker but is a real professional necessity for any therapist who needs to know what she is doing and why. It was a new facet of one's work to be prepared to communicate it to one's colleagues and the amount

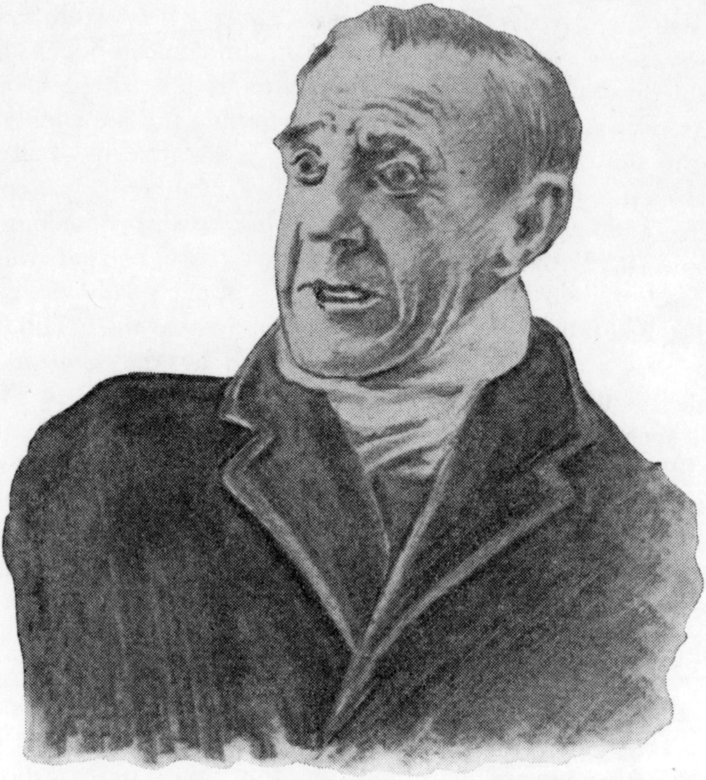

I gained from it led me much more quickly into conference participation than might otherwise have been the case.

The large conference is for many of us a method of introduction to new ideas rather than an opportunity to pursue the techniques of therapy in their most practical aspects. For this the American 'workshop', now being adopted in this country also, is the most useful. The purpose of a workshop is to explore a particular subject or technique and to involve everybody in it.

Speakers are required to give practical demonstrations on the application of the thesis they are presenting and the participants are also required to take part very actively.

I was persuaded to take part in my first workshop in the States by a very skilled and determined physical therapist who was expert in a particular technique or treatment method for cerebral palsy. The child is assisted to develop basic postures and movement in as normal a manner as possible before being allowed to concentrate on the acquisition of particular skills. Consequently the postures basic to speech as well as movement are involved.

We decided that we would each talk a little about the ideas behind the treatment but that the main focus should be on joint demonstrations with children. My colleague had previously worked at the centre where the worshop was to be held and knew many of the children. The centre was supported by one of the large and generous charitable organisations which are to be found in the States and young children were able to receive treatment without charge if the parents were of a low income group. Conditions of work were excellent and the whole place thoroughly lively and advanced.

As there were no older children there and we wished to show the school-aged child as well as the infant we had also to look outside for our subjects. I accordingly visited a large school for cerebral palsied children in the town and, mindful of what happened in Edinburgh, selected a few placid, co-operative and meek pupils to help me. They all seemed such as would not be upset by the demonstration situation nor yet relish it unduly.

However the teachers, and my colleague, all deplored the temporary absence of one child who would apparently have been just the person for my demonstration. I was assured that not only was he of considerable professional interest because of his fascinating breathing pattern, but he was exceptionally docile and easy. I agreed to demonstrate with him on sight and let me here put on record my declared intention never again to demonstrate with any child whom I have not known intimately and in all circumstances, for a long period of time.

The first part of our demonstration went very well, my physical therapy colleague getting some lovely movement patterns from the children and both of us combining to prepare them for the movements necessary for speech. I then went to the platform to give my explanatory talk which was to culminate in the appearance of the exceptionally docile and easy child. As I started on my last point I could hear the sound of bellowing, two floors up, as this same child was carried into the building.

The crescendo of sound increased as he neared the hall and as he was carried onto the platform he must have been audible two blocks away. His father, a very nice and fortunately very sturdy young man, shook his head at me over the boy's struggling body. My colleague, divided between sympathy and mirth, gesticulated loyally to the effect that if we sent him away she was prepared to masquerade as a young athetoid with an abnormal breathing pattern.

Visible on almost every face in the audience was a grin of unholy glee. They were nice amiable people but they had, after all, been there for two days being told that it was the therapist's task to encourage a child into normal channels and not allow him to exacerbate his abnormal behaviour. Now, obviously, I was to be called upon to prove it.

There seemed nothing for it but to grasp the nettle, or in this case, the struggling small boy. His father gave me a look of real feeling as I moved towards him.

'Is he in pain?'

'No, he's just mad.'

'I don't want him to leave while he is crying. If he does we will all feel bad. Can you tell him that he can go when he stops crying?'

It is well known in therapeutic and domestic circles that

whereas a young child will shout louder in response to a loud voice he may well stop to listen to a whisper. This was not a stupid little boy and he knew very well that we were planning our strategy. He paused to hear what the next move was going to be. Necessarily he paused for breath also. I told him swiftly and firmly that I was not going to hurt him and if he stopped crying and did one small thing to help me he could leave.

He opened his mouth: not, I think, to co-operate. As the first sound came out I vibrated his ribs gently which loosened up his voice and changed the strained cry to a deeper, more relaxed note. His surprise at this sound caused him to pause and then, as I did it again, to chuckle. At this point his splendid and perceptive father carried him away, leaving the audience with the sound of his chuckle and the sight of his smile superimposed on the previous adverse image. If ever I am caught in such a situation again, may I have just such a father to help me.

I have sometimes wondered whether the atmosphere of the States makes one less cautious than in England in risking oneself in hazardous situations and I have come to the conclusion that this may be so. Over there, if one has an idea, someone will back it, someone will make it possible for you to carry it out. So if one says that in order to teach effectively one must show people how to handle the children, there is a good chance that someone will collect the money and arrange for you to do just that.

It is less likely to happen in England where there is a more conservative approach to new treatment methods and where people have less cash available to put their ideas into immediate effect. But I have probably been involved in as many unnerving situations in the one country as in the other. Any situation in which one talks about one's work is potentially hazardous and a situation in which you elect to show people what you do is a risk indeed.

The department for which I now work in England is developing the use of video-tape and closed circuit television for teaching purposes and this is almost certainly the best way to show treatment. The audience does not have to be in the same room so the therapist-patient relationship is not at risk and yet the verisimilitude is unimpaired.

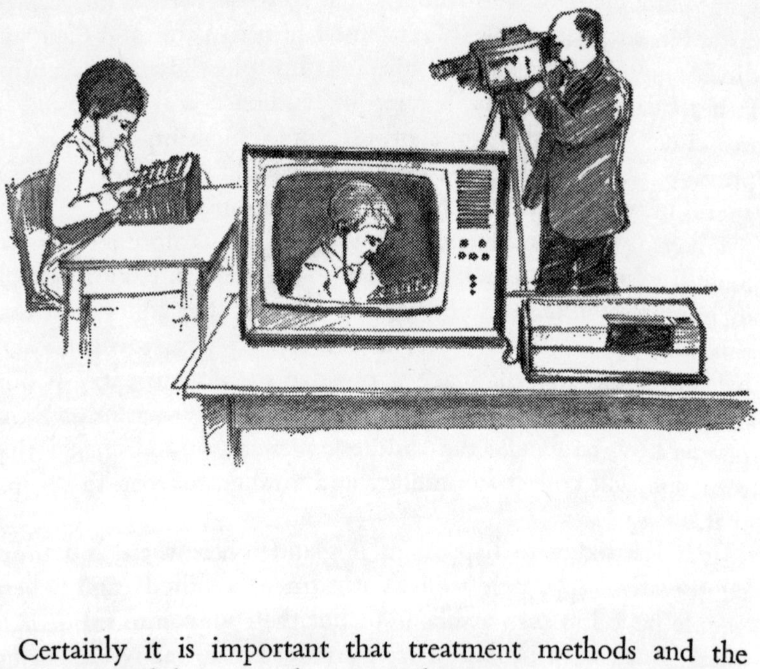

Certainly it is important that treatment methods and the application of theory to the practical situation are not only discussed but studied by a profession of therapists. It is easy to read a paper and let your words speak louder than your actions. But we advance much faster if we can together examine the whole therapy situation.

There are many benefits and bonuses that arise from any attempt to communicate with one's colleagues about therapy. After the workshop I have described, I was invited to go again to the school from which the children had been selected and spend a day working with the speech and physical therapists and teachers. This was a real pleasure.

I had forgotten something of the feeling of working in such a community but when I went back into that school with its mixture of well organised room space and children's natural mess I could have been in any special school anywhere in the world. The children showed the same postures, problems and pleasures as my children in Edinburgh and the staff had the same difficulties and rewards as we had known. Once you have worked in this kind of community you do not forget it.

I saw this point most vividly illustrated only last year by a very distinguished professor of special education, formerly an inspector of schools. We were two members of a team of three making an official visit to a speech therapy training school. As part of my duties I had arranged to visit a clinic held in a school for educationally sub-normal children. My distinguished colleague offered to drive me to the school, wait for me and drive me back.

'But what will you do in the meantime?'

'Don't worry, I shall be perfectly happy'.

This certainly seemed to be true. No sooner had we entered the building than he was greeted as an old friend by the head teacher to whom he was known only by repute and when I finished my inspection I found him tucked into the corner of a classroom as easily and effortlessly as though he had never left it. I feel something of the same familiarity when I instinctively place myself so that a spastic child in a classroom I am visiting will be able to speak to me without taking up an abnormal position; when I move into the light in the hearing impaired classroom so that the child can lip read me more easily; when I instinctively adapt my speech in the hospital so that the aphasic adult may cope with it without confusion; when I wait without effort for a stammerer to finish his statement.

Somewhere a professional unit has developed out of a person. This might perhaps have been anticipated. What could not so easily have been foreseen is that the professional expertise could have been extended into so many areas of human behaviour. And that because of this, one has a place, a point of contact and familiar territory not only in one's own country but in many other countries beside.

# II

## A RETURN TO ENGLAND AND A LOOK AHEAD

WE HAD BEEN in the States for nearly five years when my husband was offered an appointment which tempted him to return. We had reached the point where a decision had to be made as to whether to settle permanently in America or whether to come back to Britain. One cannot remain indefinitely as a visitor in another country however amicable the arrangement.

I was happy when the decision was made to return although I knew that I should miss many things about the States and not least, my colleagues and my work. But there seemed no need to contemplate a total severance. It was more than likely that my husband's work would take us back again in the future. Indeed, it was not impossible that I would get back by my own efforts.

We both looked forward to seeing our families again and to seeing our British friends in more relaxed circumstances than had been possible on our brief trips home. The Atlantic had got narrower every time we crossed it but it was still too expensive to fly back often. So far too many activities had always to be packed into far too short a time.

We contemplated our return with enthusiasm, realistically tempered with the knowledge of the advantages we were leaving behind. Our enthusiasm was certainly put to the test by the time we left. Both our departments made their adieux to us in such generous and affectionate ways that if we had not had our tickets in our pockets we might have been tempted to change our minds.

We elected to come home slowly by boat so that we could have a rest and a holiday and make the transition between one phase of our lives and another with becoming deliberation. Air travel is a fine thing but it is liable to precipitate you into one set of circumstances while the flavour of another is still with you. So we savoured our departure to the full, standing on deck as the ship pulled slowly away from the harbour at New York, drawing away from the jabby, dramatic skyline of Manhattan to steam past the legendary Statue of Liberty. My husband might have avoided the usual tourist photographs but I have no such patrician reservations. So there we are, commemorated against the background of the Statue like so many thousands of other people.

We had correctly anticipated our pleasure in our return. We had also estimated fairly accurately the things we would miss about America. But adjustment difficulties can never be entirely anticipated and there were moments when it seemed likely that we would become one of those university couples who are continually crossing the Atlantic and bemoaning on each side the advantages left behind on the other. We were glad to leave behind the violence and unrest of the States. But we missed the stimulation and positive excitement that was part of it. There was no doubt that Britain seemed cramping.

I was particularly frustrated because I was returning, full of plans, information and ideas to transfuse into the world of speech therapy in Britain and it seemed as though there was to be no opportunity for me to do so. For months I seemed to be taking my harp to a party where nobody asked me to play. When you are returning to a country which you know needs trained personnel it is disconcerting, and not pleasant, to find that you are now so well qualified as to be virtually unemployable.

My attitude was of course, both arrogant and unrealistic. I was sharing the fate of all working wives whose husband's job determines the place of the home. It was not to be expected that two splendid opportunities should burst forth simultaneously. But of course, I did secretly expect some such miracle and I champed and chafed under my professional restrictions in a highly unbecoming manner. My excess energy, which was considerable, found some outlet in knitting pullovers and amassing kitchen equipment but it was not to be expected that this could continue indefinitely.

In fairness to myself it may be said that whilst my rebellion was not gracious it was not unjustified. It is reasonable to protest against waste. Trained people should be used to advantage and in Britain they are not always so used. There is great need to consider the deployment of trained personnel in Britain generally and speech therapy is just one example.

I found considerable dissatisfaction among speech therapists as to conditions of work and considerable disquiet amongst medical and educational officers about the lack of speech therapists.

The shortage has now passed the stage of being a talking point and become a real problem. And, as happens when problems are defined, solutions are being explored. An enquiry is now under way by the Department of Education and Science to consider the profession of speech therapy. Obviously it will be some time before conclusions are reached as to how to prevent wastage and employ speech therapists to the best advantage. It is consequently unwise to speculate on what recommendations will be made. But it can only be to the advantage of our profession to be studied in this manner and most of us feel that there is now an opportunity for development that will lead to even more exciting prospects in the future . . . and better paid ones too.

I am disposed to be optimistic because it has been my experience that opportunities do appear for those that seek them. I have already described my own restlessness so it was not as the reward for patience that my next opportunity came. It was just one of those things for which one must be grateful with proper humility because it is a bonus rather than one's just deserts.

I often looked longingly at the university that housed my husband and wished that it could have been the University of Newcastle upon Tyne because that enlightened establishment boasts a degree in speech therapy, the only one in the country as yet. There I might have hoped to insinuate myself. I could not have predicted that by the end of a year I was to be busy inside those local walls as a lecturer in speech pathology and therapy.

The department to which I was appointed is long established and famous for the education of the deaf and has recently expanded to include many workers in the field of communication disorders. It reflects the growing opinion that there is no arbitrary line between hearing disorders and those of language and speech. The head of the department is a doctor of medicine and professor of audiology and in addition to the specialised and experienced staff of teachers, whose main province is in deaf education, there are psychologists and audiologists whose interests cover a wide spectrum of auditory disorders.

The activities of the department are many and varied but diagnostic work is a very important area. Full scale diagnostic clinics are held twice a week with everyone in attendance to contribute their observations and experience. There are the same kinds of problems discussed that concerned the team in the States. And there is the same attention given to following up each child's progress and trying to ensure that he receives the treatment and education that will help him to function in society.

In this department is the same spirit of interest and foresight which I found in the States but it has an extra dimension for me. It has the dimension built by a department with a long tradition of service. It was founded by someone who cared deeply about deaf people and developed by those who have been alert to the need for research and academic discipline without losing the sense of service. It is a splendid place to work.

It is an excellent thing when one is in the middle part of life to have to contribute one's mite to an established and yet expanding department. One receives the support of the structure and the stimulus of having to justify one's presence there. In a place where everything is new nothing need be accepted. In a place which is overly stable nothing need be justified.

It is good to have to examine one's own area and ideas against the critical appraisal of one's colleagues. And it is also good to have the support of their interest and suggestions. And it is best of all to see speech therapy in its broad context of communication disorders.

But I am sure that I could not have reached this point without the background of clinical experience built by the needs and demands of the children I first met. I am, of course, continually reminded of children I worked with in my first job. There was one family I often think about. They lived just down the road from the school clinic and were very steady recruits to it. At least five different speech disorders flourished in that family. Each child was speech disordered and each was speech disordered in a different way.

One or two of these children went to the special school. The others managed to get by in ordinary school with as much speech therapy as they could get. I worked hard with them, I think I helped them, certainly I delighted in them. But I think I could help them so much more now. This is not just because I have more techniques and have grown older. Techniques are only as good as the person who is using them and being older is no guarantee of enlightenment. I could help them more because more is known.

If those children came to see me now I would be better able to see their speech disorder in relation to the whole area of language learning. I would consequently be able to evaluate their language abilities in a way more helpful to their teachers. And I would run less risk of skating over something that could cause educational difficulties later on.

I remember being asked at the first parents' meeting of the

Spastics Association in my county borough at what age I would start working with a spastic child. I only hope my answer has long been forgotten because it was 'Five'. Five months would be a closer estimate now. This was not just a mistake on my part, nor was I merely ignorant and naïve. At that time we did not know enough of the sequence of normal speech development to appreciate at which point we should be intervening.

But it is no good thinking complacently of one's increased knowledge. I have no doubt that we will all be blushing just as much over our present ignorance in twenty years time as we now are over our past.

The College of Speech Therapists has now been established for twenty-five years. It is, and should be, proud of the high standard of professional competence it has developed and maintained but, as the field of communication disorders opens up, new methods must be evolved to meet its demands. This means that our training must be adapted and almost certainly extended. We want to see postgraduate courses available in universities for speech therapists. And we want these speech therapists to be given extra pay for their additional qualifications.

In America there is stratification within the profession and the titles of speech pathologist, speech therapist and speech correctionist are used to denote degrees of qualification as well as areas of interest. In Britain we have not accepted divisions within the profession. It was probably necessary at first to establish the profession through its basic qualification. But now that this has been achieved we need to find ways of ensuring that senior people in the profession will be able to put into useful and profitable effect the experience they have gained and that people with specialised knowledge will be able to make full use of it.

At the present time a senior speech therapist can have her work counteracted by the arrangements or views of those who know very little about communication disorders. Not only is she discouraged but her patients do not receive the help which they need. We would like to see the status of our senior people raised so that they can contribute much more effectively to the overall organisation of the profession.

The status of the profession would, of course, be considerably enhanced if the training were carried to degree level. A door has opened with the setting up of the degree course in the University of Newcastle upon Tyne, in 1964. Graduates from this course are recognised by the College and encouraged to join it. If other university courses are started, as is hoped, the College will doubtless adopt a similar policy towards them. We may reasonably expect to see a modification of the role of the College from the sole controller of training to the regulator of professional standards and conduct.

The College of Speech Therapists elects its council from the membership and so many of us have been poacher turned gamekeeper and gamekeeper turned poacher at various stages of our careers. When not serving on Council we protest about the lack of activity in vital areas and the apparent inertia of the governing body. When serving on Council we protest about the unrealistic demands of the membership and its apparent inertia ('Why will people never answer questions, read notices, inform us of change of addresses' etc.'). This is all rather normal I should think in a government of a profession by its members.

But outsiders cannot know and even insiders cannot really appreciate the amount of care and thought that goes into it all. There is no effort spared to see that the practising members of the profession have all the encouragement and knowledge that can be given them. A most successful provision is the setting up of refresher courses and there are also area meetings and discussion groups so that no-one need be cut off from information and opinion. We certainly do not want to lose these core activities and have the profession in a state of individual enterprise that will prevent the exchange of knowledge and the mutual support of its members.

But there is, of course, a more convincing reason for the necessity to co-ordinate the profession under one professional body. We are working with vulnerable people. Our patients have lost, or not acquired the means of communicating easily with others. They are at the mercy of anyone who will offer them hope however expensive that hope may be to realise.

Papers are quick to publish new 'cures' for stammerers and for speech disordered children. Individuals and organisations are quick to exploit suffering. The parents of handicapped children are intensely vulnerable to this exploitation. No loving parent, or guilt ridden parent of a handicapped child can ignore an offer which suggests that the child can be made normal.

It is for professions to protect vulnerable people from exploitation by offering them a body of personnel who will themselves be protected from unrealistic assumptions by their training just as they will be led into further knowledge by their continuing exposure to new developments. These trained people must be registered with an organisation whose officers can send information to any concerned official or worried relative. There is no substitute for such a body.

So the continuance of the College is vital for the maintenance of a service just as the development of the profession is vital for the increase of that service. The fuller the participation of its members the more satisfactory its activities are likely to be.

Students coming in to the profession now will be given much more information and more guidance in how to use it than was possible in my days as a student. We need many more recruits and I am confident that we will get them.

When I was teaching at the Central School we received an application from a prospective student warmly supported by her headmistress. The headmistress concluded her remarks by saying that 'she is not in the least deterred by the prospects of an arduous and ill paid career'. This letter quite delighted me and I quoted from it soon afterwards at a careers conference of teachers which I had been asked to address. I went on to say that the profession was no more arduous than many satisfying and valuable areas of work and that the poor pay would certainly be remedied. Moreover, I stated with conviction, these were the only two things that could possibly be said against a job which offered so much in terms of public service and personal satisfaction.

As I relaxed after these words a familiar figure approached me. She offered me a piece of paper and said how glad she was that I had found something to keep me busy and occupied for such a long time. The paper revealed a ribald poem composed by me when its possessor was the teacher of the fifth form Latin class and I was an inattentive, scribbling pupil.

At this point in time I do believe myself to have been extremely lucky to have been kept so happily occupied in my work. But I do not believe myself to be unusual in this respect. Many others will have been lucky too. If there are other jobs that offer more, then it is for other people to evaluate them.

One cannot be both judge and advocate and my allegiance has been long since pledged.

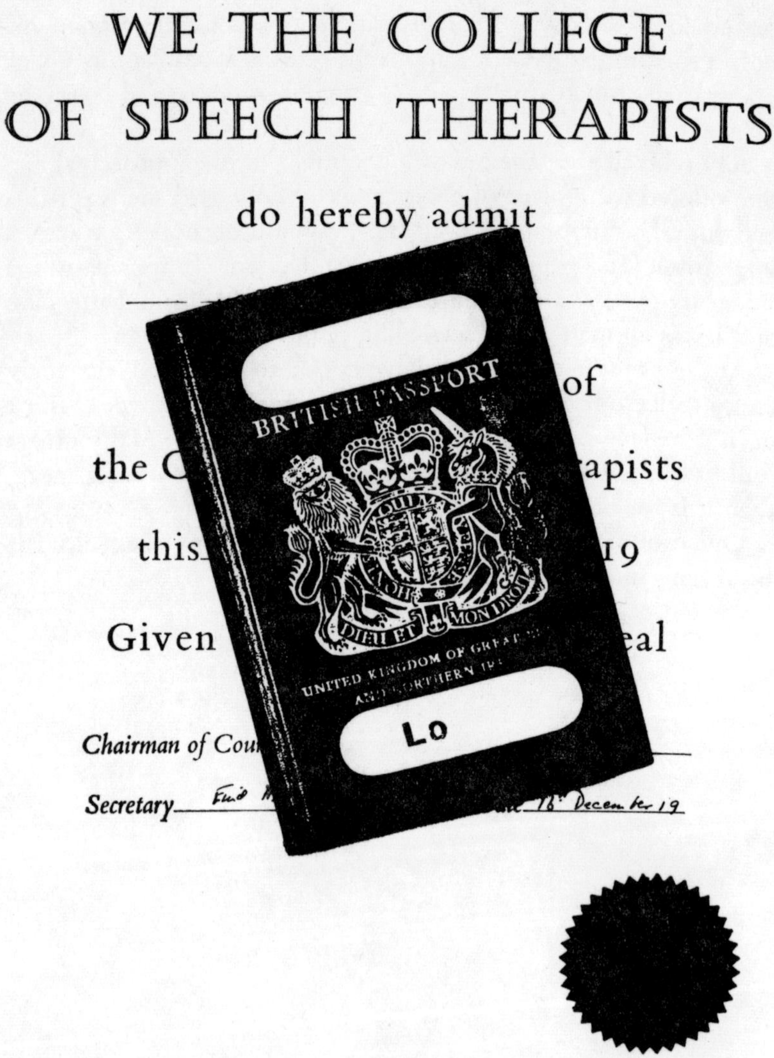
WE THE COLLEGE
OF SPEECH THERAPISTS
do hereby admit
of
this
19
Given
BRITISH PASSPORT
DIEU ET MON DROIT
LO
Secretary

# APPENDIX

## THE COLLEGE OF SPEECH THERAPISTS

The College of Speech Therapists is a legally incorporated body and membership is open only to those who hold its diploma or whose qualifications are recognised to have equivalent status. It was formed in 1944 to bring together all practising speech therapists in Great Britain and to organise and conduct examinations which would ensure that new entrants into the profession had attained a recognised standard of knowledge.

In addition to providing information about training, the College has a number of informatory leaflets on speech disorders which can be sent on request to parents, teachers and other interested people. Their present address is:

The College of Speech Therapists,
47 St. John's Wood High Street,
London, NW8.

It is suggested that people who are interested in the history and development of the profession of speech therapy and the College in relation to this should read:

*A History of Speech Disorders*
by Margaret Eldridge
published by E. & S. Livingstone.

The following training schools submit students for examinations by the College of Speech Therapists:

The Birmingham School of Speech Therapy,
North Birmingham Technical College,
Bonshaw House, 868 Bristol Road,
Birmingham 31.

The Edinburgh School of Speech Therapy,
7 Buccleuch Place,
Edinburgh EH8 9LW.

Elizabeth Gaskell College of Education,
School of Speech Therapy,
Hathersage Road, Manchester 13.

Jordanhill College of Education,
School of Speech Therapy,
Southbrae Drive, Glasgow, W3.

The School for Disorders of Human Communication,
86 Blackfriars Street,
London, SE1.

Sub-Department of Speech,
Department of Biology, Leeds Polytechnic,
Calverley Street, Leeds LS1 3HE.

City of Leicester College of Education,
Department of Speech Therapy,
Scraptoft, Leicester LE7 9SU.

The Oldrey-Fleming School of Speech Therapy,
84a Heath Street, Hampstead,
London, NW3.

West End Hospital Speech Therapy Training School,
59 Portland Place,
London, W1N 3AJ.

There is at present only one University Degree Course in Speech Therapy. This is the degree of B.Sc. in Speech.

The University of Newcastle upon Tyne,
Sub-Department of Speech,
46 Leazes Terrace,
Newcastle upon Tyne, 1.